All about me

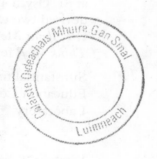

Nelson

Schools Council 'Health education 5-13' project

This project was established by the Schools Council in 1973 at St. Osyth's College of Education, Clacton, Essex and has devised two teacher guides for children in the 5–13 age range:
All About Me for the early years of schooling (5–8)
Think Well for the middle years of schooling (9–13)

Substantial financial support was also provided by The Health Education Council and the Transport and Road Research Laboratory.

Project Team

Director : Trefor Williams
Deputy Director : Ian McCafferty
Evaluator : Marilyn Stephens
Research Officer (also Project Disseminator) : Vaughan Johnson
Advisory Teacher, seconded by I.L.E.A. : Clyte Hampton
Advisory Teacher, seconded by Cardiff L.E.A. (part-time):
Paul Nelmes

All about me

Teacher's guide for the early years of schooling (5–8)

Thomas Nelson and Sons Ltd
for the Schools Council

Thomas Nelson and Sons Ltd.
Nelson House   Mayfield Road
Walton-on-Thames   Surrey
KT12 5PL   UK

51 York Place
Edinburgh
EH1 3JD   UK

Thomas Nelson (Hong Kong) Ltd.
Toppan Building 10/F
22A Westlands Road
Quarry Bay   Hong Kong

Distributed in Australia by
Thomas Nelson Australia
480 La Trobe Street
Melbourne   Victoria 3000
and in Sydney, Brisbane, Adelaide and Perth.

First published 1977
ISBN 0-17-423067-2
NCN 11-1HU-0379-04
NPN 10 9 8 7

Acknowledgements

The project team wishes to express its gratitude to all those who have assisted in the preparation of this guide, in particular to Peter Tomlin for his illustrations; to Joan Bliss and Rose Roberts for their invaluable criticisms and ready suggestions, and to all those teachers, too numerous to mention individually, in Cardiff, Essex, London and Oxford who contributed to the early work of the project; and to those in Cardiff, Essex, London, Oxford, Newcastle, Nottingham and Sheffield whose trial of the materials in the classroom played such a major role in the development of the guides. The project team is also grateful to Jennifer King, of the London Hospital Medical College Dental School and Dr John Beal, Campaign Director, Remember Your Teeth Campaign and Senior Dental Officer, Avon Area Health Authority (Teaching), for taking on the task of revising the sections on dental care for this edition.

Phototypeset by Tradespools Ltd, Frome, Somerset
Printed in Hong Kong.

Contents

General introduction

It will soon become obvious to the reader as he or she glances through the pages of this guide that our interpretation of the word 'health' is very wide, embracing as it does not only physical health and hygiene but also the emotional and social facets of human life. It follows that our interpretation of health education is also broadly based so as to include those planned experiences which we believe will benefit the physical, emotional and social lives of children.

Because we have defined health education so widely, its aims would seem to coincide exactly with the accepted aims of 'mainstream' education. Both seek to equip individuals with knowledge, skills, values and attitudes which will help them cope successfully with their present and future lives. Indeed, so exactly are the aims of health education and education itself matched that it might appear to be unnecessary, even extravagant, to think of either as separate from the other. In practice, however, much health education teaching occurs as an incidental addition to other work instead of as a planned part of a child's school experience; sometimes it is tacked on as an afterthought, sometimes omitted altogether.

The function of this guide is to draw the attention of teachers to the kinds of experiences which can be provided for young children in school. These experiences will, we believe, enrich them and increase their capacity to deal effectively with 'health' matters. Some of the ideas and teaching strategies will be familiar while others will be less so but we have, with the assistance of groups of teachers in different parts of the country, arranged them in a form which we hope will be helpful to the classroom teacher.

I

Some of the ideas offered for consideration might appear to some teachers to be not very relevant to the lives of young children, but our reason for including them is based firmly upon two well established observations:

i   That children's out of school experiences are far wider and more varied than some teachers acknowledge.

ii That children's values and attitudes towards certain topics of health related behaviour (such as smoking) are already forming at an early age. Such values and attitudes are very important, in the long run, to the development of patterns of health behaviour later in life.

The importance of the infant and lower junior school in the formation of children's attitudes to themselves and other people, their habits and general social development is an established fact. This guide seeks to offer help and practical suggestions which teachers might find useful in encouraging positive attitudes and meaningful development.

Synopsis of the chapters

1 *Finding out about myself*
The opening chapter lends itself to work with younger children. It looks first at the body and the senses and then leads on to the inner self of feelings and emotions. It can be used therefore as a springboard for work in several of the following chapters, and also provides a beginning for the self concept theme which is threaded at different levels through the subsequent chapters.

2 *How did I begin?*
This chapter deals with different types of birth, with pregnancy and with human sex and the care of young babies. It could logically follow from work in the previous chapter, although there are a number of alternative suggestions for ways in which this subject could be introduced. It is stressed that work of this kind should be put in its natural context, and that teachers should be aware of just how much information children of different ages have and need to know.

3 *What is growing?*
Growing in all its aspects is considered in this chapter – not just physical growth but also the growth of abilities, the

development of interests and the increasing responsibility in the school and at home.

4 *What helps me grow?*
The chapter begins by stressing the important love and care element of growing, and then moves on to look at the more obvious elements of exercise, rest and food.

5 *Looking after myself*
After considering some of the more traditional health education areas, such as washing, dressing and looking after teeth, most of which might seem more appropriate to younger children, the chapter goes on to deal with disease and medicines, and finally with the problem of smoking.

6 *Keeping safe*
The material is divided into sections on roads, outside places and home and school. In the road safety section the work is in three stages, the level of vocabulary and activity getting higher as children get older. There is a strong emphasis on practical work at the roadside.

7 *Knowing about others*
This provides a balance with the first chapter, which is largely self centred, whereas this concluding chapter looks outwards at other people. It starts in school and moves towards friends and then families, keeping in mind the ideas of belonging, sharing, helping, being responsible and understanding about rules.

Using the guide

Planning a programme for the early years of schooling

The guide can be used in many different ways, but our hope is that it will provide a framework for and a stimulus to staff discussions concerning the relevance and place of health education in the school curriculum. Experience has shown that the impact of this work is greater when considered as an integral part of the school curriculum and when a sequential pattern of work is planned to occur throughout the school life of children. Teachers will be well aware of the importance of repeating work at different times to coincide with levels of development and interest of children. They will also be aware of the value of adopting a variety of approaches so as to enhance the learning process. Road safety education, for example, should be seen as a continuous pattern of work which occurs throughout the early school life of children and we have suggested three distinct stages which can be adapted by teachers to their own situations. Similarly each chapter contains suggestions for classroom work which could be developed in a sequential way to coincide with the particular needs of children at different ages.

While recognizing the need to spread the work fairly evenly over the years of early school life, teachers nevertheless often wish to give particular emphasis to certain parts of the work at different times in a child's school career.

Outlined below is the attempt of one school to organize the sections of the guide to cover a four-year period. It must be re-emphasized, however, that such a method of organization should reflect the needs and interests of particular children, teachers and schools and should remain as flexible as possible.

A suggested four year programme

Year 1 *Myself* – as much of chapter 1 as seems appropriate
Together in school – first part of chapter 7
Road safety–stage one – first part of chapter 6
Looking after myself – first part of chapter 5

Year 2 *Finding out more about myself* – latter parts of chapter 1
How did I begin? – the whole of chapter 2
My friends – second part of chapter 7
Looking after my teeth – second part of chapter 5
Road safety–stage two – second part of chapter 6

Year 3 *What is growing?* – as much of chapter 3 as seems appropriate
Looking after myself – third part of chapter 5
Road safety–stage three – third part of chapter 6
Keeping safe outside – fourth part of chapter 6
My friends – second part of chapter 7

Year 4 *What helps me grow?* – as much of chapter 4 as seems appropriate

4

Looking after myself and others – fourth part of chapter 5

Smoke and me – the last part of chapter 5

Home and families – the third part of chapter 7

Keeping safe at home and school – the last part of chapter 6

Working across chapter boundaries

In a subject such as health education there are inevitably many cross references between chapters. Special signposts (marked ♦) are used to indicate points where these are particularly appropriate or relevant. We realize that not all teachers will wish to follow our particular organization of the material and within the context of a 'centre of interest', 'topic', or 'project' approach there will obviously be work which crosses many chapter boundaries. It is our hope that teachers will not be inhibited by the artificial boundaries created by division of the material into chapters but will instead use the book as a flexible planning guide. As an illustration of how teachers have used the guide in this way we include two flow charts, but again emphasize that these are only two of many different possible approaches.

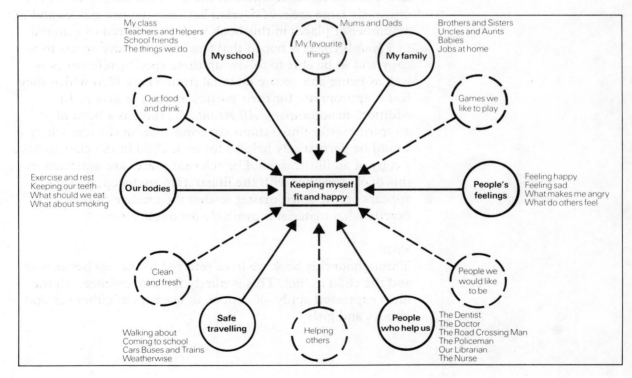

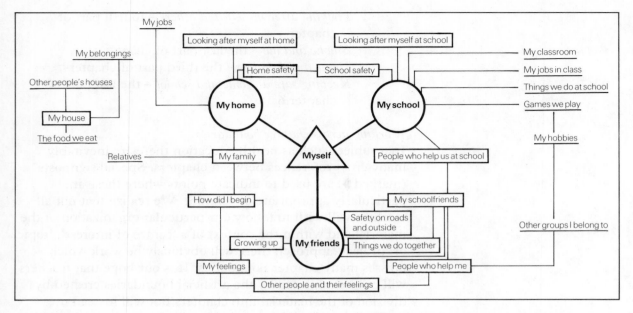

The *Schools Council Health Education 5–13* project has resulted in the production of guides for teachers of two age ranges: *All About Me* for teachers of the 5–8 year age range and *Think Well* for teachers of the 9–13 age range. There are obviously large areas of overlap between the two guides and in a number of places in this book we have referred to material in *Think Well*. It is hoped that teachers will have access to a copy and so be able to follow up these specific references as well as being able to use material from *Think Well* which they feel is appropriate for their particular class or group. In addition, to accompany *All About Me*, there is a book of 16 spirit master illustrations covering areas in the text where it would be particularly helpful for each child in the class to have a copy of an illustration. The relevant places are indicated in this book, together with the illustration (reduced) which appears on the spirit master so that the teacher can see exactly what material is available for duplication.

NOTE
Throughout this book we have referred to the teacher as 'she' and the child as 'he'. This is purely for convenience. All the ideas expressed apply, of course, to teachers of either sex and to boys and girls.

1 Finding out about myself

Introduction

This chapter should be seen as a springboard for those
following: it offers a possible starting point, particularly for
the teacher of early or middle infant children. The purpose of
the work suggested is to provide children with opportunities
to explore their physical and emotional selves within the
secure and trusting environment of the classroom. It is also
hoped that the teacher herself might develop a sharpened
awareness of those processes, of which she and the school
are part, which contribute to the image that children
develop of themselves.

Our earliest forms of exploration are concerned with
developing awareness of our own bodies. During the first
year of life, a child learns to discriminate the 'me' from the
'not me'. Through touch, smell and sight he learns to
recognize boundaries between himself and the world outside,
and it is from this early awareness of his body that his idea of
'self' develops. He becomes conscious too of feelings 'inside' –
of hunger, fear, frustration and anger. The image of himself
that he builds up is reinforced and developed by what he
sees reflected back at him from a mirror. His mirror image
tells him whether he is tall or short, black, brown or white
skinned, blue, green or brown eyed.

The image of himself which a child develops is not merely a
mirror representation of his physical self, however; it is
composed also of ideas about himself which he perceives to be
reflected back from people who are close and important to
him – parents, guardians, teachers. To the young child these

important adults appear large, powerful and privileged. They make things happen and provide for his needs; they seem, to him, to enjoy total freedom of action and complete self confidence. The reflections he receives from them tell him whether he is valued or not valued, good or bad, loved or not loved, liked or disliked.

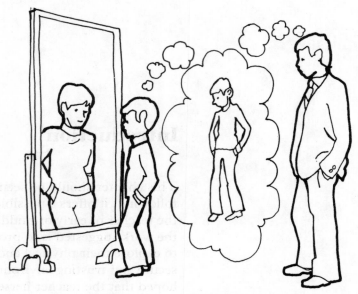

Real image reflected from the mirror: 'I am tall and strong'

Perceived image reflected from a 'significant' person: 'Teacher thinks I am a poor weak thing'

Through self-exploration and social interaction with people of importance and significance to him the child builds up a complex image of himself called his *self concept*. His self concept determines how he expects others to behave towards him, and influences the way he behaves towards others. If a child has no experience of love and respect it is difficult to extend them towards others.

On coming to school, children have already developed many different perceptions about themselves and their abilities. These perceptions can be thought of as invisible tags which accompany them everywhere, and which to them are as real as true mirror images. When the tags are of a generally negative nature, it is possibly more damaging than a physical handicap; the most insensitive of us make allowances for physical disabilities, but a child with a bruised or damaged self perception is often overlooked.

8

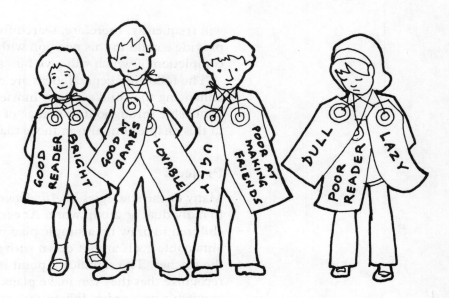

The child's self concept will determine his response to many situations – does he come to school predisposed to achievement and success, or to under-achievement and failure? Does his experience at school support or undermine his belief in himself as a valuable person? Some of the child's perceptions about himself are, of course, based on reality and cannot be changed, so they must be faced and accepted as part of the process of developing and maturing. Other perceptions may be 'distorted' reflections.

The teacher as an adult of some importance will exert considerable influence on the child's self concept. The child's expectations of his own capabilities may be set too high or too low, and the teacher is then confronted with the problem of matching the child's expectations with her own. A child may, in order to safeguard himself, set his expectations so high that failure is *certain*, rather than attempt work whose outcome may be *uncertain*. On the other hand, setting his sights to a low standard will bring success but will not extend the child.

The ethos of work in the early school years is such as to develop in the child a sense of achievement by learning new skills and mastering different materials. The work done during this period of development is influential in improving or confirming the child's idea of himself. Many things are, however, impossible for the five and six year old – there may be, for example, little or no scope for satisfaction in the completion of reading or number assignments. The teacher

9

will frequently, therefore, search for ways in which she can provide a child in this position with suitable activities, the completion of which will give him a sense of achievement.

The following general ideas are offered with a view to enhancing the child's idea of himself and should be seen as applicable throughout the range of strategies offered not only in this chapter but also in those that follow it.

Projects

Many of the strategies in *All About Me* lend themselves ideally to individual or group work. At certain times it is fruitful for children to draw up a simple plan of a project in which obtainable goals are set down with the help and guidance of the teacher. The significant point is that children should recognize that they can make plans themselves. They will inevitably encounter difficulties and even disasters but with help and guidance these can be overcome, to the immense satisfaction of the children.

Projects can be chosen from a wide variety of activities – at school, in the classroom, in the playground, doing a particular piece of work, working with certain children, or at home, doing jobs, being helpful, tidy, kind, obedient and punctual.

Plans of action

Similar ideas and methods may be used to make a group or class plan in which the children will need to co-operate in determining their goals and attempting to carry out their plan. Class or group plans need to be prominently displayed and will clearly require longer to complete than individual projects. They might be related to preparation for a presentation at a school assembly, making group or class booklets, making models or pictures or other joint activities. It is important, however, that children should know clearly what part each individual plays in the activity and to have an opportunity to discuss such contributions. The teacher's knowledge of the children in her class will be of inestimable value in helping to shape such plans.

Trying something new

Children enjoy repeating activities which have given them a measure of success but they can also derive pleasure and confidence from mastering a new activity or skill. The strategies which follow offer many ways of giving children new experiences and opportunities to attempt new activities and skills. At certain times it would be advantageous to high-light 'trying something new' – this would give an opportunity of discussing realistic and unrealistic aims.

It is clear then that the teacher plays a role of considerable importance in being able to influence not only the child's self concept but also his capacity to relate to others, and his emotional health. *Finding out about myself* is an exercise devoted not only to the exploration of the child's *physical* self but also to his 'feelings' self. It is also likely that some of the strategies suggested will give the teacher a greater insight into the social interaction of her class, as well as the behaviour of individual children.

Looking at ourselves

This is intended to summarize the activities which will provide a common starting point for young children to begin their individual investigations. Start by stressing characteristics common to all children, making use of the vocabulary they will need when talking about themselves. Replies to some of the following questions will provide a good beginning to the work.

How do we find out about things?

We can see . . .
We can hear . . .
We can smell . . .
We can taste . . .
We can feel . . .

What can we do?

. . . with our eyes
. . . with our ears
. . . with our noses
. . . with our tongues
. . . with our hands
(Don't forget winking, wrinkling of noses, curling of tongues,

waggling of ears, shaping with fingers, etc.)

What do we do?

We eat, we sleep, we run and walk.
We work, we play, we laugh and talk.
    The children can make rhymes and riddles, and match
sentence cards such as: We can smell . . . . . . with our
noses, relating the activity to the correct part of the body.

How do I know what goes on around me?

Work about the five senses could now turn to an appreciation
of how they are important to us in everyday situations. A
great deal of language work can be done in the form of
recognition games and exercises.

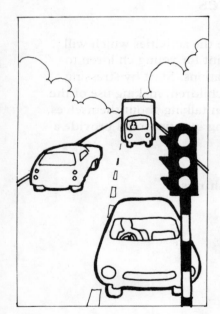

What do my eyes tell me?

Using a drawing like the one shown, flannel-graph figures,
pictures or the scene outside the classroom window, point out
that our eyes can judge distance, size, shape and colour.

What do my ears tell me?

The children will be able to distinguish typical sounds and
certain degrees of volume and pitch. Use a tape recorder to
try 'animal' sounds, 'kitchen' sounds, 'school' sounds,
'playground' sounds.

What does my nose tell me?

Ask the children to guess what is in 'smell-bottles'. Try
coffee, onions, etc. What words can we give the 'smells'?

What does my skin tell me?

Discussion centred on a class weather chart could readily
lead on to how our skin detects and reacts to change in
weather conditions.
       Warm   Windy   Wet   Cold   Itchy

What does my hand tell me?

Put different items into the 'feel-boxes' to encourage descrip-

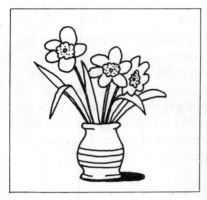

How can we tell if these are plastic flowers?

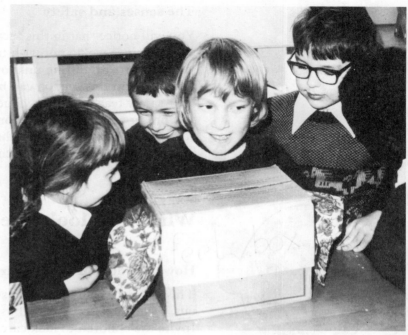

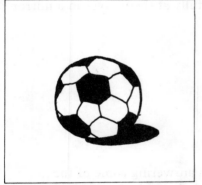

How can we tell whether this football is ready to play with?

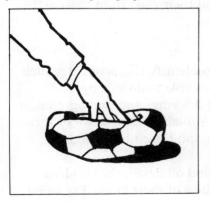

tive vocabulary. You could try a toothbrush, a sponge, some jelly, some fur, sandpaper, etc.

As an alternative to using the 'feel-boxes' ask the children to touch or handle articles behind their backs, under a table or when blindfolded. Remember to point out that by preventing them from seeing you are stopping them from using their most valuable sense.

– When we can't see what do we do instead?
– Do we need to see to answer the 'phone or listen to the radio?
– Do we use only our eyes when we watch television?
– Can we tell where someone is by the sounds he or she makes?

Some teachers have developed this theme, as a result of the children's interest, by discussing with them blindness and what it must feel like to have to depend upon the other senses. 'Centres of interest' and small projects have been built around such subjects as *Guide dogs for the blind* and *The use of braille*.

At this stage the emphasis should be upon the way the senses complement each other to provide the body with a balanced pattern of information. As each sense is used this pattern should become clearer.

The senses and safety

You will notice that in this section the 'taste' sense has been avoided since we do not wish to encourage children to experiment with tasting unknown substances. Much of the work done in this section can be seen as ground work for later safety teaching. The value of developing keen senses for self-preservation should be borne in mind, as in seeing a car coming, hearing a wasp, smelling fire and so on. Further information will be found in chapter 6 (*Keeping safe*).

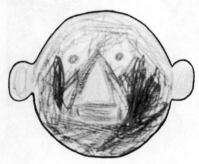

What do I look like?

How well do you know your face?

This should provide an interesting exercise in looking, finding out, recording, drawing and using descriptive vocabulary. Invite the children to look carefully at themselves in a mirror and suggest some questions.
- Where are my ears?
- What shape is my nose?
- What colour is my skin?
- What colour are my lips?
- What colour is my hair?
- What colour are my eyes?

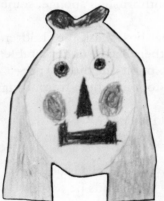

Rogues Gallery
After looking at themselves and answering some of the relevant questions children might be invited to draw a picture of themselves to be mounted in a 'Rogues Gallery'. See if they can identify others in their class from these self portraits.

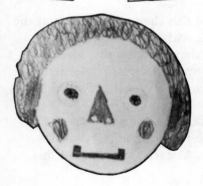

'Identikit' pictures
Older children could attempt to identify characteristics such as shape of head or face. It is possible to do this by encouraging children to look at drawings and photographs of people. If a polaroid camera is available, choose two or three different shapes of face, photograph the children and cut round the shapes.
   As a result of this concentration on detail, the children should be able to make up pictures of their faces. Try using

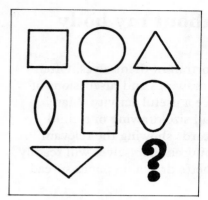 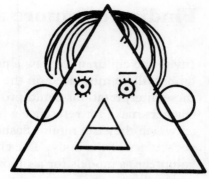 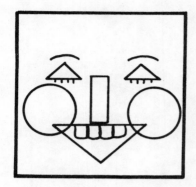

basic shapes to stick on duplicated outlines until they have a
complete identikit picture of themselves.

My mouth
- How many teeth?
- Any coming through?
- Any missing?

Are my eyes . . . ?
- Blue, grey, brown, hazel, black, green

Is my hair . . . ?
- Black, brown, red, green, fine, coarse, thick, thin, straight,
  curly, crinkly

Profiles and Masks
Other interesting details can be derived from discussion about
individual profiles of heads, while some teachers have
encouraged children to make face masks as a development of
the identikit idea.

Shape of hair also lends an interesting dimension to an
understanding of individual appearances.

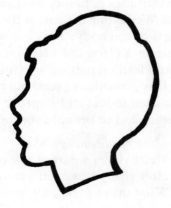 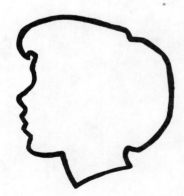

Finding out more about my body

Invite the children to draw a portrait of themselves. Often limbs will be misplaced on the drawings and discussions of these interpretations could prove a useful activity. Many teachers make for reference a full size drawing of a child on which they can mount flashcards showing the relevant vocabulary of the body. The children themselves will readily volunteer as models for a silhouette drawn on paper spread on the floor.

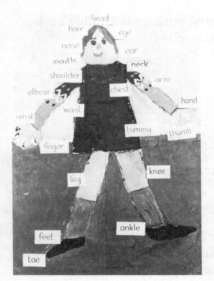

My shoulders
- How many ways can I move them?

My chest
- What happens when I breathe deeply?
- When I breathe out?
- What's beating in there?

My tummy (stomach)
- Is it full or empty?
- When does it rumble?
- Does it ever ache?

My body alphabet
Arm (ache)
Back (bruise)
Chest (cough)
(Doctor, Dentist)
Ears
Face   Finger
Gum
Head   Hand
(illness)
Joint
Knee
Leg
Mouth
Nose

This is a good point to discuss the differences between boys and girls, about which children will be naturally curious. The amount of knowledge that the children already have on this subject will vary enormously and will depend very much on attitudes at home, whether a child has brothers and sisters, etc. We favour the use of the correct vocabulary to describe parts of the body. This is discussed in the introduction to chapter 2 (*How did I begin?*) and indeed work in this section could lead on naturally to much of the work in chapter 2.

It is possible for teachers to make simple work cards for children to test and improve their knowledge about their bodies and to provide vocabulary exercises.

Finding out about my body   *Card one*
- Write down a part of the body with eight letters.
- How many ways can you move this part of your body?
- What other parts of your body are attached to it?

The rest of me
- How far can I turn round from my waist while sitting down?
- How many joints can I find?
- How do my arms work?
- What is the smallest thing I can pick up with my toes?
- What is my footprint like?
- Why do we wear shoes?

Teachers wishing to provide opportunities for older children to develop a more detailed understanding of their bodies will find the unit, 'Ourselves' from the Schools Council project, *Science 5–13* of particular value at this point.

 Further ideas about how the body works will be found in chapter 4 (*What helps me grow?*).

Handicapped people

In discussion with children about their bodies, questions about handicaps are often raised, indeed it is not uncommon for children suffering from various handicaps to be present in the class, sometimes in wheelchairs. If this is the case, teachers need to be aware of how willing such children are to talk about their handicaps and how sensitive they are about them. If a handicapped child were particularly sensitive about his disability, a good way to introduce the subject would be to invite an adult with a similar handicap to talk to the class. (The teacher should first make sure that he or she is used to talking to young children.)

It may be that a handicapped child in the class is quite willing to discuss his physical disabilities, in which case this is a useful way to introduce the subject. Perhaps the teacher could start by asking the handicapped child how his disability came about. It could be explained that people can become handicapped in several ways: by being born with the handicap; by being injured or through an illness. Teachers need to explain that handicapped individuals are unable to do the kinds of activities which the majority of children are able to take part in, due to lack of control, strength, or mobility in one or more parts of their body. It will probably be the case that the handicapped child does other activities while the rest of the class is doing games, PE, movement, etc. As a result, unusual skills may be developed and this fact should be emphasized to the other children.

Children are always very interested to learn of the ways in which handicapped individuals often overcome their disabilities. One interesting development is for children to consider the Paraplegic Olympiad which is held, like the Olympic Games, once every four years. Some schools also arrange for older children to visit schools for the handicapped in order for them to see what handicapped children are capable of doing.

Other things which make me 'myself'

Things I like

Give the children an opportunity to talk about what they like. They could record and illustrate their lives in a variety of ways, for example by making a montage after cutting out pictures they like. Older children will be capable of sorting their responses under headings – possibly separate pages in a booklet:

Games I like to play with	Things I like doing by myself
People I like to play with	Places I like to visit
Toys I like to play with	Things I like listening to
Food I like for breakfast	Clothes I like to wear
Food I like for dinner	Stories I like to hear
Food I like for tea	Songs I like to sing
My favourite game	My favourite food My favourite song

Groups of children could make posters to show their favourite games, foods, animals, toys, etc., using cut-out pictures or drawings, each child to contribute one item to each poster and to append his name.

– Are there things we all like to do?
– Are there foods we all like to eat?

Things that make me feel

Teachers have found simple drawings such as those at the top of the opposite page may be copied easily by children when they are writing about or illustrating an experience they have had. Other teachers have found it more useful to have available complete pictures of children because, they maintain, posture is able to convey a greater meaning than facial expression alone. Suitable examples are given on sheet 1 of the *All About Me* spirit master book.

Spirit master sheet 1

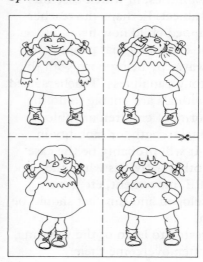

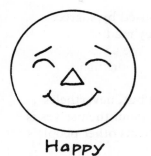

Happy

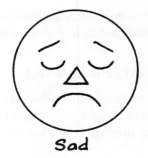

Sad

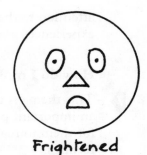

Frightened

Angry

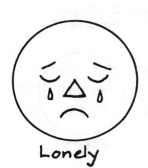

Lonely

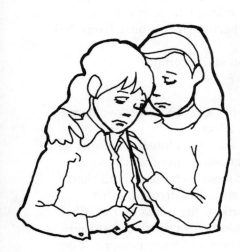

The topic may be introduced by reacting to a spontaneous show of emotion, using a story such as *Mr Happy* (see Resources list page 121), reading a poem or displaying items which will produce emotions – sweets, a favourite story book, a broken toy or spoiled picture. Several class booklets could be made from the resultant children's writing and drawing.

The things which happen which make me feel

The children will be eager to share their experiences with each other by talking, drawing and writing about them. Many opportunities for expanding this expression of emotions exist, particularly in the field of drama. For example, a group of children could relate an experience and explain it to another group who then act out the situation. This benefits both groups. Alternatively, the teacher might present a situation to a class which the children can then mime. Older children, for example, might, in the course of a movement lesson, be told that they have just received some bad news (or good or exciting news) and they are to find a sympathetic friend with whom to talk about it. Ask the children, in groups, to act out this situation.
- Does the sympathetic friend really listen to you?
- Is he really interested?
- What does it feel like?
- How can you console a friend in such a situation?
One feature of 'Finding out about myself' is that this work will help children to understand that their feelings are not unique. It is important for them to understand that other people have feelings too and although this facet of the work is developed in greater detail in chapter 7 (*Knowing about others*), this is a useful place to introduce it. Story times are particularly useful for this, and teachers should draw

attention to the emotions and feelings aroused by shared experiences as described in any stories they read.

How do I make other people feel

 This theme is also developed in chapter 7 but, nevertheless, an important part of children finding out about themselves is for them to realize how their behaviour affects other people's feelings.

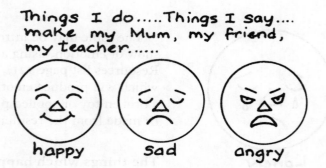

Younger children might be given the opportunity of acting out or making pictures of how they affect others. For example, if the children are in pairs, they might take it in turns to behave in ways that will elicit a particular response from their partner.
– How does he behave when you start crying?
– How can you make him laugh?
– Can you make him scared?
Ask them to describe how their faces, bodies, movements change in order to have such an effect.

Teachers will need to discuss with the children reasons why their behaviour evokes such reactions from others.

Older children might like to choose a character and then either write a poem or act out a situation involving this character. Give them time to think of the behaviour of other people which caused their emotion before they act out their feelings by gesture, facial expression and body posture. They should then have an opportunity of explaining to the rest of the group the situation and behaviour of others which led to such strong feelings.

Choose from :
Angry Alan or Ann
Jealous John or Jean

Frightened Fred or Freda
Friendly Frank or Francis
Sad Sally or Simon

Some teachers have developed this theme to introduce the idea that each of us can behave in such a way that we change someone else's feelings in a positive manner.

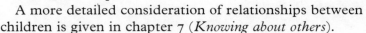

Older children can develop this idea to include thought about how they can intervene positively in a social situation. They can discuss with the teacher how to recognize such a situation, what sort of behaviour is required of them, and how their behaviour might have consequences for others, for example in the situation illustrated on sheet 14 of the *All About Me* spirit master book (see page 109).

- How can I tell when somebody is lonely or feels out of things?
- How can I help?

A more detailed consideration of relationships between children is given in chapter 7 (*Knowing about others*).

Concluding activities

Many teachers have felt a need to pull together the many strands and ideas in this chapter by some kind of concluding activity which gives children an overview of the work undertaken. In some cases this has been accomplished by displaying a selection of relevant pieces of work in a confined area so as to facilitate a discussion and review of what the children have found out about themselves. Many teachers have also found these ideas useful as a framework for a play or a school assembly. Others have asked their children to complete such a review in a more formal way by having them write or draw an answer to the question, 'What have you found out about yourself?'

Many of the ideas expressed in this chapter are, however, picked up again in later chapters and the things which children have discussed about themselves form obvious, interesting and ongoing links with such work.

2 How did I begin?

Introduction

As many teachers will realize, the work suggested here could with some advantage be incorporated into that of the previous chapter. There are also links with chapter 3 (*What is growing?*) and the first section of chapter 3 might introduce this chapter. One of the hoped for outcomes of the work contained in the early chapters is the development amongst children of a 'matter of fact' and wholesome attitude to themselves and their bodies. Such an attitude is reflected in their willingness to ask questions about sex and reproduction, and needs to be matched by the teacher's willingness and capacity to answer. The atmosphere which a teacher creates in a classroom is crucial to the learning which takes place there, particularly within the context of human reproduction and sexuality.

Young children come to school with some understanding of their sexual identity as represented by their ideas of what it is to be male or female. These ideas arise out of a variety of experiences but are, largely, connected with their relationships with adults who are important to them. In obvious and not so obvious ways adults expect boys and girls to behave differently and children learn to act in accordance with these expectations. Children identify with adults of the same sex and, learning from the ways in which adults of opposite sexes interact with each other, copy attitudes and postures in a variety of situations. Attitudes at home to many sexual situations – nudity, exposure in the bathroom or toilet, on

23

television programmes, in photographs – will colour children's attitudes.

It must be remembered that young children are extremely curious about their own bodies. At home and at school children are encouraged to inquire into and become aware of their environment, but are not given similar guidance or support when they investigate the nearest and most puzzling factor – their own body. It is a normal activity for them to explore their own genitals and to take pleasure in doing so. These activities must not be wrongly interpreted as abnormal displays of sexuality, and teachers should be prepared to meet such situations when they occur.

The process of socialization itself then has given all children a sex education of some kind by the time they start school. It is as well to remind ourselves that such influences do not suddenly cease but, on the contrary, become more intense as children get older. Newspapers, magazines, radio, television, films and, later, peer groups all contribute significantly to the social climate – a climate of which children become increasingly aware as they get older.

We see a clear role for the teacher in this respect: to help young children cope successfully with these influences. This is not to say that sex education should be force-fed to children but rather that we should ask ourselves what experiences we can give children which will help their self-development and self-acceptance and so enable them to better understand and cope with their own sexuality.

Many schools use a carefully thought out programme of work in this field, including in it a variety of approaches, and covering different aspects during the child's school career. These programmes frequently involve discussions with parents before starting the work for the first time, sometimes showing them the teaching materials to be used.

There are, we believe, several important ideas which can be successfully pursued and developed with young children, as a result either of following the interests and questions of children or of seizing upon opportunities which arise spontaneously. In each case however the teacher will need to think carefully about how such a topic might be developed, the kind of questions which children are likely to ask and, more important, the kind of answers she should give.

The ideas which we believe should form the core of such work are:
- Living things come from living things

- Like comes from like
- Human babies (and other mammals) grow inside their mother before they are born
- Both men and women are needed to make babies
- Babies grow in different ways after they are born and have to be cared for by adults

In the course of the work suggested children will ask 'awkward' questions and a few examples are given below. Possible answers to such questions are given primarily as an indication of the general level of answer that might be suitable.

Some typical questions which may arise and suggested answers

– Where was I born? Where do babies grow?
(A special place in the mother's tummy called a *womb*.)
– How long do babies stay inside?
(The mother has the baby growing inside her for about nine months. For this time she is called *pregnant*.)
– Did I come from an egg?
(Yes, the egg was inside your mother.)
– How do the eggs start growing?
(Father's seed [*sperm*] needs to join the mother's egg [*ovum*] before it can grow.)
– Where does the sperm come from?
(The sperm comes through the father's *penis* from his *testicles*.)
– How do babies feed (or eat) inside?
(They get food from their mother's tummy. It is dissolved and transferred from the mother's blood to the baby's blood. It is passed to the baby along a special tube called an *umbilical cord*. The place in your tummy where the umbilical cord was attached is called a *navel*.)
– What is being born? How does the baby get out?
(Muscles inside the mother's tummy push the baby down the mother's *vagina*.)
– Why is the baby upside down?
(So that the baby can come out of the mother [be born] more easily.)
– How do babies get inside? How are babies made?
[This question is dealt with in detail on page 31.]

In their responses teachers will need to give some thought to vocabulary as this will have considerable bearing upon the

25

children's understanding of what is being discussed. Generally there is a tendency to favour the use of the correct vocabulary (penis, vagina, sperm, umbilical cord, etc.) but teachers do nevertheless have to remind themselves that children come to the classroom with different and often idiosyncratic sets of words related to the private parts of their body. This vocabulary is closely related to regional and social background and should be treated with respect even if such words are not to the liking of the teacher herself. The teacher will have to consider how best such an individualistic vocabulary can be gradually exchanged for a more public and common language so as to facilitate later discussions about sexual reproduction and other pertinent matters. The use of suitable books and other aids will be of considerable benefit here, and some are suggested in the Resources list (see page 122).

Another matter demanding some consideration and thought is that concerning references to 'family'. We consider it undesirable that this area of work should be discussed without relating it to family life in general. Children will, naturally, particularize so as to use their own experiences of family life, and teachers need to consider the effect this might have when presenting and developing the work. This matter is discussed in greater detail in the introduction to chapter 7 (*Knowing about others*) and teachers are invited to read that section in conjunction with the present introduction.

In many ways it is a pity that work of this nature is labelled 'sex education' because it can so easily result in a teaching form which tends to segregate the work from other activities being pursued in the classroom. Such a label also heightens feelings of anxiety amongst teachers who would feel more comfortable integrating the ideas and concepts within the general work of the class. The teacher is encouraged therefore to use the ideas which follow in any order or sequence which seem logical and appropriate to her particular situation.

Living things come from living things

There are, of course, many ways in which activities might be sparked off:

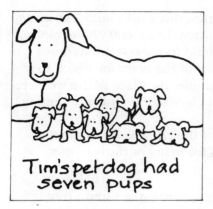

Tim's pet dog had seven pups

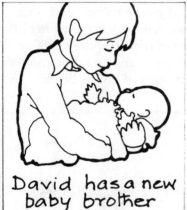

David has a new baby brother

News items
The subject might arise as a result of children's 'news' items such as the birth of a new pet or an addition to the family.

Stories
Many of the books available to children centre upon family life and the activities of its members. Often these stories include the coming of a new baby or the birth of a puppy or kitten. Such work could lead, without much difficulty, to a general discussion about babies and their needs. In the secure familiarity of such discussions teachers might ask:

Where do you think you came from?
This question might well be asked in the course of a general discussion about babies and their needs. In addition to this being a potentially humorous exercise, we do feel that it is important that the children should be encouraged to express their ideas of where they came from. Any myths should be aired at the start of this section so that misunderstandings may be more readily corrected.

Other work
Work done in other chapters, for example in Chapter 1 (*Finding out about myself*), Chapter 3 (*What is growing?*) or Chapter 7 (*Knowing about others*), could well lead into this topic.

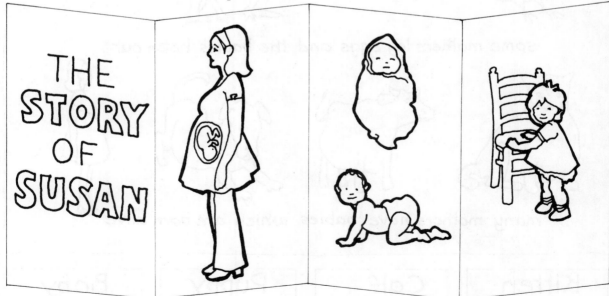

THE STORY OF SUSAN

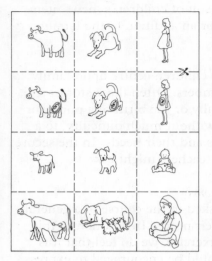

After the introductory activities, this work could lead on to case studies of one or more children, using real photographs where possible. Such a study could introduce children to a shared vocabulary for those parts of the body for which they have no common name, for example, the place where we were before we were born – a special place in the mother's tummy called a *womb*.

The illustrations on sheet 2 of the *All About Me* spirit master book can form the basis for many of the activities suggested in this chapter.

Some babies hatch from eggs, some are born alive

Children are fascinated by birth and young babies, and some will already be aware of different ways in which the young of several species are 'born'. A display of pictures, drawings or posters of different creatures and their young could be used to stimulate work on the two different ways of giving birth

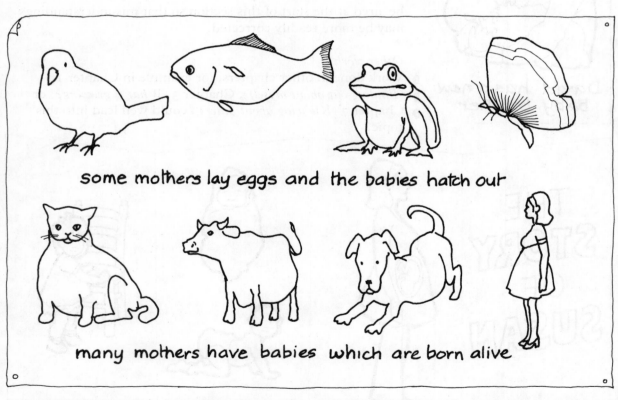

some mothers lay eggs and the babies hatch out

many mothers have babies which are born alive

| Kitten | Calf | Puppy | Baby |

mentioned above. The children could cut out photographs of different animals, or draw their own pictures, and stick them on posters or into their books.

Discussion about how babies are born might lead naturally to a consideration of the fact that 'like comes from like'.

Like comes from like

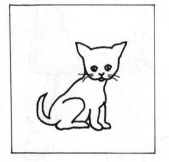 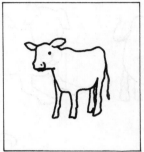 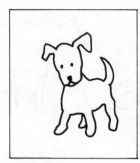 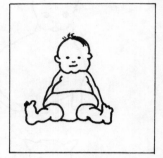

Which mother?

At this stage the children will be keen to match the young with their respective parents. A simple matching game using 'animal-family' cards could be devised, and the posters used before could now be used to show the baby beneath its parent.

Needless to say this activity lends itself not only to the development of a general vocabulary but to many other activities involving sorting, number work, art and creative writing.

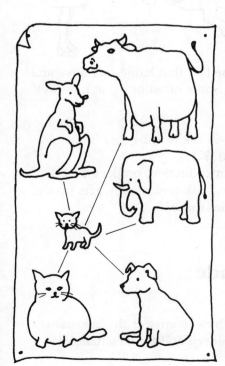

Some schools have produced a frieze of animals, including humans, and their young and this has provided an excellent background for classroom displays of children's work as well as being a stimulus for further investigations.

Whose baby?

An example of a drawing or poster posing this question is shown.

Name the young

The children should choose pairs of flashcards and relate them to the correct photograph or drawing displayed, or to one drawn by them.

29

Babies grow inside the mother before they are born (mammals)

All these mothers are expecting babies. If we could see inside their wombs this is what we would see.

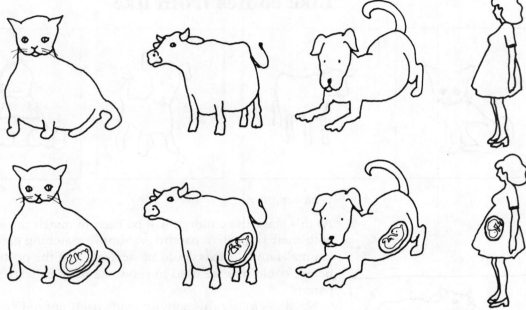

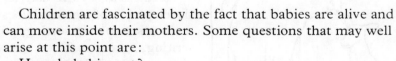

Children are fascinated by the fact that babies are alive and can move inside their mothers. Some questions that may well arise at this point are:

How do babies eat?

Why are babies upside down in the womb?

How long are the babies inside?

(Answers are suggested in the introduction, on page 25.)

Occasionally an older child will ask how a baby gets inside in the first place, 'How are babies made?'

How babies are made

Teachers will have to consider how to answer this question in terms best suited to their children and to the situation in which it arises.

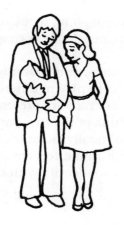

It is likely that the children will already have reached the conclusion that both male and female are involved, in some vague and unspecified way, with the making of babies. There is a need for the teacher to clarify, in terms comprehensible to children, *how* both men and women are needed to make babies. It is obviously important that teachers think not only about what they will tell children but also about how they will say it.

Essentially an answer to such a question might include reference to the man's seed (sperm) meeting and joining with the woman's egg (ovum) which then grows gradually over nine months into a baby. Children are fascinated by the sequence of growth and the size of the baby at the various stages. Many teachers have shown pictures and photographs which illustrate these stages while others have found that sectional models are of great value in helping children to understand the growth process. In a wider context many teachers feel that keeping pets in the classroom on a regular basis can provide a natural background for and stimulus to their discussions with young children on this subject.

Teachers and parents become particularly anxious when considering how to explain the act of procreation in a way which has meaning for children. Such explanations need to be simple, sympathetic but frank and might include a description of how when a man and woman care for each other they sometimes cuddle up close together which they both very much enjoy. Sometimes the man places his penis into the vagina of the woman and after a while the seed passes through his penis into the woman where it might find its way to the egg.

There are several books and items of audio visual material which can be of particular use to both teachers and children and a list of these can be found in the Resources section (see pages 122 and 123).

How babies are cared for

Who gives babies what they need?

It is of great importance that before delving too deeply into this subject teachers consider any 'unusual' family back-

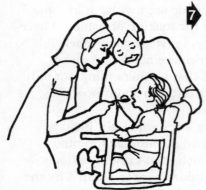

grounds and the possible effects of investigating them. This area of work is considered in much greater depth in chapter 7 (*Knowing about others*).

Families in general, brothers and sisters, grandparents, uncles and aunts may have special roles to play in different social situations and where differences of race are present. It is important that children do not think of the two-parent nuclear family as being the only 'right' family situation. The result might be that some children would feel abnormal or inferior as well as finding it difficult to identify with the examples given.

What do babies need?

Food and sleep
Discuss how much, and how often, young babies need feeding or are asleep.

Love and protection
This must be central to any discussion about babies – their helplessness and dependency on adults.

This section provides a link with work in chapter 4 (*What helps me grow?*).

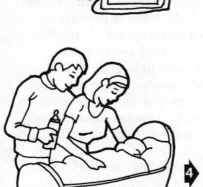

What do babies eat?

Adults care for babies

These points should be raised in discussion, by the teacher if not by the children:

- Milk is the food of all babies that are born alive.
- Babies can suck as soon as they are born.
- Human babies suck milk from their mother's breasts.
- Bottles, with a teat shaped like the mother's nipple, are sometimes used to feed babies.

Mothers feed their babies

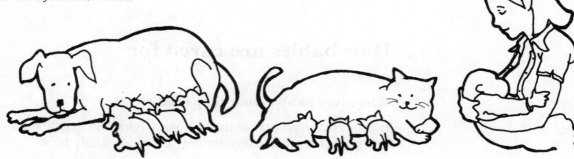

How quickly do they grow?

- Why does it take so long for a baby to grow into a man or woman?
- What happens as we grow up?

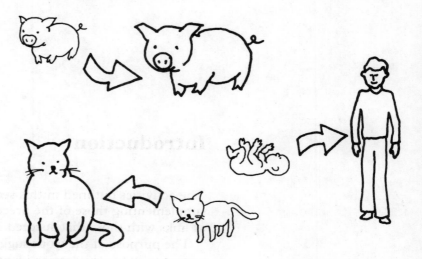

In what ways do they grow?

Children could select other children from several different age groups and draw and mount silhouettes of them for purposes of comparison.

Older children could be given the opportunity of finding out how much height and weight variation there is within specific age groupings.

 This work on growth provides a series of links with the following chapter (*What is growing?*).

Nicola
6 months

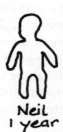
Neil
1 year

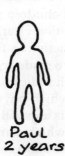
Paul
2 years

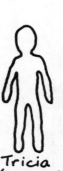
Tricia
6 years

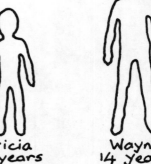
Wayne
14 years

3 What is growing?

Introduction

The activities outlined in this section should be seen as supplementing those of the preceding two chapters and also as links with those that succeed it.

The purpose of the work suggested is both to provide an opportunity for children to identify the ways that growth occurs in the physical, emotional, social and intellectual spheres and also to enable them to understand that physical growth is predictable and that it is unique for each individual. Each class has children of different sizes and builds, with varying interests and abilities; it has its leaders and followers, its quiet and noisy members, those who are shy, afraid, noisy, quarrelsome, happy or contented. The teacher's specialist knowledge of her group of children can be applied towards assisting the individual child in those ways which make the best possible use of his unique blend of abilities. The work done in first schools particularly is largely directed towards encouraging and shaping the child's development in as many different directions as possible.

Serious consideration is given by teachers to the *physical growth* of children since size, stamina, physical skills and co-ordination clearly limit the suitability and range of possible activities for the young child. Height and weight checks are made regularly at most schools for record purposes, as a rough indicator of the child's growth rate. The variety of ways in which physical growth can be measured and recorded makes this a useful exercise and produces much display material which can demonstrate stages in or comparisons of growth for all to see.

Much attention is also paid to *intellectual growth* – to the acquisition of the knowledge and skills which will provide the basis for further development. Educational objectives may be expressed and intellectual achievements measured; marks, graphs, progress charts can show progress (or lack of it) to the child, his friends and others.

Presenting far greater problems for the teacher in terms of content, method and organization, however, is the *social* and *emotional* growth of children. Most teachers would accept that they should attempt to establish which children have difficulty making friends, which are shy, afraid, frequently upset and so on, and that they have a certain responsibility to help children overcome these problems. Yet although these dimensions of growth are possibly the most important, the opportunities for the children to actively explore, recognize and cope with their emotions and those of other people are often missed. The potential interest of the child in new groups, making new relationships, reacting to his new status or responsibility may be wasted unless his attention is carefully drawn towards this aspect of his growth.

In the course of this work, opportunities will abound for comparisons to be made between individual children or groups of children, younger and older, in the family or at school. However, it is most important to bear in mind the possibilities of invidious comparisons within these groups. Many graphs and charts purporting to show growth level can be damaging in that they publicly type the child as 'small' or 'average' or 'unable to tie shoe laces' yet without specifying that this was in one growth dimension within one group of children at one time. Comparisons between children undoubtedly serve a useful purpose, as also do averages and rank orders, yet in this work the individual child's position relative to his own growth pattern is much more important. It must be remembered that the rate of growth is dependent upon a variety of factors such as inherited characteristics, diet, exercise and rest, and that there are liable to be changes in this rate, shown by the occasional growth 'spurt'. Reassuring those children who are worried by too much or too little growth at any one point will be an important part of the teacher's role.

Helping children to see ways in which they have progressed over time will also reassure them. This might well involve teachers in considering facets of 'progress' – for example, ability in games, social interaction, capacity to work alone, the use of books, etc – which they might not have considered before. Sometimes teachers see such little progress over time that the operation can become depressingly negative. It is important at that point to consider seriously the implication such work might have for the individual child as well as for the teaching. The danger is, of course, that the child's sense of his own failure will be reinforced, this being the last thing that the teacher had intended.

This section, then, assumes that the child has found out a lot about himself and he is eager from this knowledge of his own position to look backwards to the younger brother or sister at home, his own photographs, discarded clothes or outgrown toys, or perhaps to the children in the classroom he has just left. In addition he will anticipate the activities in which he will soon be tall or strong enough to take part: he may be aware of some attitudes, reactions or behaviour which he is now capable of classing as 'babyish'; he may wish to belong to new groups of friends and take greater responsibility for his own activities – in other words he is aware of the fact that he is growing but he will need guidance and reassurance to help him come to terms with the different ways in which this is happening. The work in this chapter may stem from several starting points:

- As a result of questions or work arising from chapter 1 (*Finding out about myself*) or chapter 2 (*How did I begin?*).
- A young baby or brother/sister coming to school.
- The annual weighing and measuring recording session.
- Starting a new activity, keeping pets, going swimming, etc.
- Moving to a new classroom or a different part of the building.

The starting point will in some measure determine the types of approach, of which three main groups are suggested here.

Individual scrap books or folders

The children can make their own books using real photographs of 'me the baby', drawings, pictures, children's 'interviews with mother', old belongings, etc.
Some titles suggested are:

How I grew up
Me growing
We grow
Growing is

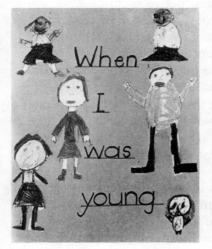

Group comparisons

The class can be divided into groups, each group to research, record and summarize information by concentrating on specific aspects of growth. The information should be put together to present the whole picture and to give a balanced view. The following breakdown could be used:

- *Our size and shape* (height, weight, surface, space filled)
- *Our interests and abilities* (games, 'favourite . . .', hobbies)
- *Our responsibilities* (to family, friends, school)

Case histories

These might be made of two or three individuals. They would be researched in depth, the individuals being chosen for their apparent similarity or difference. Photographs, tickets, postcards, articles of clothing and so on can be used. Some titles suggested are:

My passport   My police record   The group file

How my size and shape change

This section provides an excellent link with the previous chapter (*How did I begin?*) or, as some teachers have shown, serves as a useful introductory phase to it. Teachers generally have used considerable flair in their efforts to stimulate the imagination of their children as some of the following items will illustrate.

I have grown out of . . .

To encourage the concentration on comparison with their previous size the children could be asked to collect items for a display: outgrown clothes and shoes, articles they used as a baby, photographs of themselves as a baby and so on.

. . . baby things

A high chair, cot or pram could be brought into school and become the focus for discussion. The children could 'measure' the furniture they used when they were younger against their present school chairs/tables.

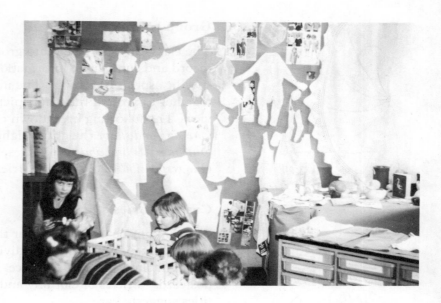

In the early stages show relative sizes by placing objects side by side and using 'bigger than' or 'smaller than'. Later on, introduce more precise vocabulary – wider and narrower, taller, shorter, longer, higher, thinner and thicker.

I am taller now or I can reach further than before

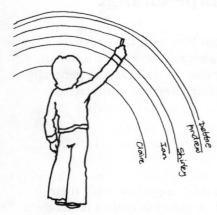

As a variant on the standard ways of height measurement, ask each child to draw an arc on the wall. They must take it in turns to stand upright with their feet on a marked spot for the curves to run parallel. Seven children with the requisite colours could devise a method for constructing a rainbow sequence.

These marks can be left on the wall for several months and the children can then repeat the exercise and see how much further they can reach.

– Are there other ways of finding out whether we are taller now than a year ago?

I can jump this much

Once the 'reach height' and 'jump height' have been marked, the children can compare not only the height from the floor or bottom of the blackboard, but, more important, the difference between their own two marks. Those who have the biggest gap between these two marks can jump the most, although they may not actually jump the highest.

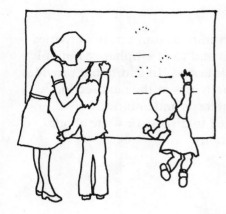

Much of the work that is done in studying growth patterns and rates ends up in the form of graphs and charts showing the tallest, fastest, strongest, or heaviest child at the top. Various procedures could be devised to compensate for this tendency by providing achievement situations for the smaller child who is less able at jumping or skipping. Older children should be capable of resolving some of the more interesting relationship questions shown below.

I can curl up into a smaller ball

Those who can tuck themselves into the smallest possible ball will score more in this game. The circular grid can be used in many ways for games but also serves a useful measuring function:
- Does the tallest child make the largest ball?
- Does the shortest make the smallest?

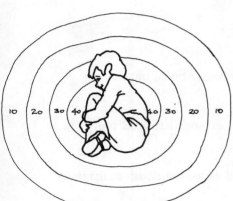

I can crawl under (do the 'low jump')

- Can I make myself thinner and flatter?
- Is the shortest child also the thinnest?

How I fit into the pattern of growth

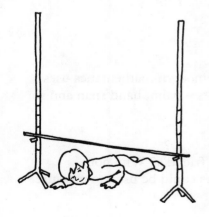

So far the activities suggested have avoided direct comparisons between children and have concentrated instead on the uniqueness of growth patterns. However, the children will certainly be aware of the differences in size between themselves and their friends of the same age. An opportunity for comparisons which allows several children to be 'tallest' and several 'shortest' within any one class could be made by using group investigations.
- How tall are the children on my table?
- How far would we reach if we lay head to toe?
- How heavy are we separately? As a group?
- Is the tallest person also the heaviest?
- Who wears the largest plimsolls? (Surface of foot.)
- Who wears the largest gloves? (Surface of hand.)
- Who has the 'biggest' head? (Distance round head.)

Me growing

This section provides an opportunity to sum up the activities concerned with physical growth and to re-emphasize not only its predictability but also its uniqueness. In addition it provides a useful starting point for the activities in the next section which deals with developing interests and abilities.

Children might be encouraged to discuss or write about their present and future aspirations.

- I used to _____ then
- I can _____ now
- I hope to _____ soon

First I was a baby
tiny boots, bonnet, socks, jacket . . .

Then I was a toddler
walking reins, romp suit, toys, boots, shoes, hat . . .

Now I am a young boy/girl
school bag, books, hat, boots, more sophisticated tools . . .

Next I shall be a teenager
larger clothes, long trousers, make-up, handbag, magazines . . .

One day I shall be a fully grown man/woman
largest clothes, tools, kitchen equipment . . .

More measurement

Much measurement practice in modern mathematics uses parts of the child's body for units – palm, hand span and so on.

- How many 'hands high' is _____ ?
- Is my answer the same as my friend's? Why not?
- What other parts of our bodies could be used to measure with?

Older children can be extended much more in this section since they are able to use standard units. However, it is easy to concentrate too much on height, length and width to the exclusion of other more interesting measures. Hands and feet offer a great deal of scope for more detailed investigation:

My hand, my brother's hand, my dad's hand

outlines
cut-outs
handprints
fingerprints
surface area
width of palm
length of finger
thickness of nail
  – Is the right one equal to the left?
  – how much can I hold? (use clothes pegs, seeds, newspapers)
  – how much water does my fist displace from a full container?
  – how much plaster do I need to fill a clay mould of my
    thumb?
  – what is the smallest object I can pick up and hold?
  – what is the largest ball I can pick up from on top and hold?
Similar comparisons might be made between various other
parts of the body such as:
circumference of head
circumference of neck
length of forearm
length of lower leg
size of feet
  Older children might even consider the ratio of various
parts of the body to each other and compare them with those
of other people.

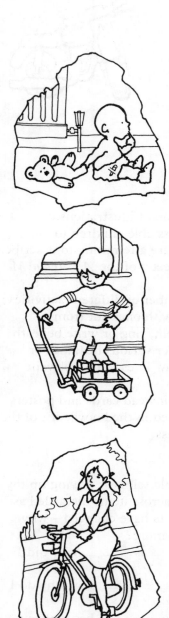

My interests and abilities develop

The children will know that some of their classmates can
read or write better, run faster or in other ways demonstrate
their interests and abilities. The value of stressing *individual*
growth patterns in a variety of skills, interests and abilities
is clear in the case of the undersized, overweight, or 'under-
achieving' child. For the 'normal' child it may also serve a
useful purpose in illustrating areas where further development
could take place!

As we grow older our interests change

A series of snapshots, slides, catalogue pictures or even
cut-outs from comics would serve to start the discussion.

I can do many things now

I can . . .
jump higher, run faster, walk further, dance, skip, ride . . .
a scooter   . . . a tricycle   . . . a bicycle   . . . a motorbike!

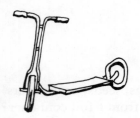 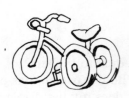 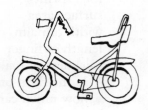 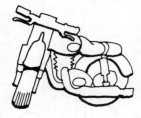

Spirit master sheet 3

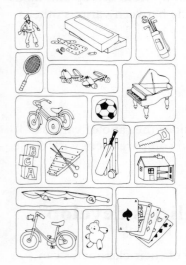

Baby's? Mine? Grown-up's?

Children could be shown a collection of illustrations of objects, some of which may help less able children to remember games or toys that they are attempting to describe. A suitable collection is given on sheet 3 of the *All About Me* spirit master book.

This sheet can be used for a number of different activities. Children could cover the pictures with ones cut from magazines or catalogues, colour them, ring or write beneath those they like most, put them under various headings or write in ME, BABY, DAD and draw lines to the relevant pictures.

Teachers may well prefer to use instead cards and posters which they themselves have prepared in the knowledge of the interests of the children in their class.

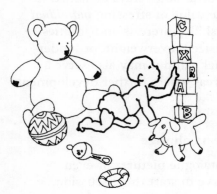

Things I used to play with
In the course of collecting for jumble sales, or tidying up toy cupboards, the children will come across items discarded as 'babyish'. Discuss how their interests have changed – why don't they play with those toys any more?

– My favourite toy used to be _____ is _____ why did I change it?
– My favourite book used to be _____ is _____ why do I like this one?
– My favourite television programme _____ has it always been the best?

- My favourite food used to be _____ is now _____ have my tastes in food changed?
- Food I dislike _____ have I ever tasted it?

Invite children to show three ways in which their interests have changed since starting school. Invite them also to show three skills they possess now, that they didn't have before they came to school (reading, writing, dancing, etc.). These activities could involve writing, drawing or mime.

 This work is developed in greater depth in Chapter 4 (*What helps me grow?*).

What things can grown-ups do which I can't do?

What would I most like to do out of these?
- Where did you get the idea?
- Why do you want to?
- Do you think you are going to change your mind?
- What would you like to do which you are not allowed to do?

Much fascinating information can be gained about the way children view the world of adults and their place in it. This work could lead on to discussions about trying something new.

I would like to be able to _____
_____ drive a car, train, bus
_____ pilot an aeroplane
_____ knit a jumper
_____ bake a cake

I would like to be _____
_____ a filmstar   _____ kinder
_____ a postman   _____ smaller
_____ a milkman   _____ larger
_____ a teacher   _____ better at art

Trying something new

Discuss the things that the children would like to do which they have never done before. Many of them will set their aspirations too high, offering completely unrealistic responses. Discuss the full list of both realistic and unrealistic aims in the hope that the children themselves will sort out which new activities they really could do and would be prepared to try. This process in itself is most useful, yet even more important is to follow it up by discussing the likely reasons for the success or failure of the attempt.

- What would you like to do that you have never done before?
- Could you really do that?
     No (discuss, discard, start again)
     Yes (plan how to set about it)
- How did you feel?
- Was it what you expected?
- Will you try it again?
- Now try something else.

My responsibilities grow

No matter what stage the child has reached, an earlier stage can be indicated where there was greater dependency for basic needs – satisfied by mother, father or possibly teacher.

When I was very young I needed someone to . . . feed me . . . dress me . . .

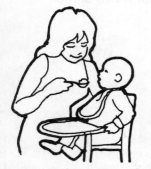

What did I do when I was hungry and thirsty?

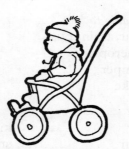

How did I keep warm?

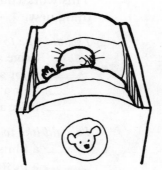

Why didn't I walk? How did I move about?

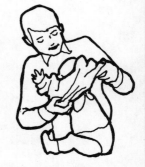

Where did I sleep? How did I get to bed?

Now I am older I know how to . . . I know I should . . . do I?
Ask the children to list, portray in pictures, mime, or merely tell of the many actions they can now perform for themselves. Ask if they enjoy doing them and if not why should they do them?

- clean my teeth regularly
- dress and undress myself
- clean my shoes – tie the laces
- take care of my clothes and kit
- put myself to bed without fuss

Point out their increasing responsibility for using these capabilities.

 This section provides a link with chapter 5 (*Looking after myself*).

Jobs I can now do in the classroom and at home

As children get older they will readily appreciate that younger children need more attention and cannot be given as much responsibility. Discuss with them their growing responsibilities and ask what jobs they are now capable of doing at home and at school.

- tidying up my desk
- helping to give out materials
- clearing up after craft
- librarian
- monitor for _____
- tidying up my toys
- answering the telephone
- caring for pets
- cleaning my room
- looking after baby brother

 This provides a link with work in chapter 7 (*Knowing about others*).

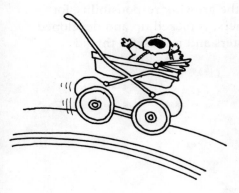

What could I do?

Using pictures or dramatic scenes discuss what a baby could or would do and what an adult would do. After this, discuss with the children what they could and would do. Again, many children will offer completely unrealistic responses and these should be discussed and the children encouraged to suggest actions which are within their capabilities. Encourage suggestions of methods of helping, working together and taking responsibility. Exploitation of actual classroom/playground situations will be of even more value.

What should I do?

A series of dramatic situations could be presented and discussed, and the results depicted in various ways – by painting, written work or a completed mime performance. The sequence would be to present the children with the scene and ask what the participants and witnesses should or would do.

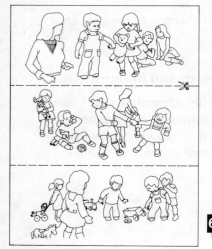

Get the children to act the parts or record them as a child in the situation, as an observer, or as a grown up. Drawings such as those given on sheet 4 in the *All About Me* spirit master book could be used as a starting point or else the children could be presented with situations such as the following examples:

● A new girl has joined the class this morning. She looks very sad and lonely.
● It's John's turn on the swing and he's been waiting for ages. At last the little girl gets off but the swing knocks her over.
● Baby Lynette is asleep inside the house. Someone notices some smoke coming out of the window . . .
● A young child falls over a mat and grazes his knee . . .
The last two situations would provide a link with work in chapter 6 (*Keeping safe*).

Concluding activities

It would be particularly useful if in discussion with the children the teacher could make a summary of the work attempted in order to emphasize that growth occurs not only in a physical sense but also in terms of interest and responsibilities – including social responsibilities.

This last point, concerning the growing responsibility for looking after ourselves and others, is picked up and developed in each of the succeeding chapters and is a useful thread which links them together.

4 What helps me grow?

Introduction

This chapter follows on logically from those preceding it and offers supporting ideas and activities on the theme of growing. It must be stressed that the capacity to 'feel' for others is an important component of growing. Children, and adults too, grow emotionally and socially in a loving and caring environment. The capacity to understand such feelings requires as much consideration as other aspects of growing and, therefore, it is important to include discussions of love and care when considering *What helps me grow?*

Other activities in this chapter are concerned with the part played by exercise, rest and food in helping growth and each section is prefaced by its own brief introduction.

Initially, suggestions are made for a fairly general approach which might be particularly suitable for younger children while later in each section activities are included for older infant and younger junior school children.

What do we need for growth?

Discuss with the children what growing means and relate back to their previous work concerning the different ways in which we grow. One effective technique for stimulating discussion would be to pose carefully chosen questions and encourage the responses to be given in mime, by role-playing or in pictures. Some examples of questions are given below:
– How long could you sit perfectly still? What happens?

- What do you feel like in the morning if you go to bed very late?
- What do you feel like if you have missed your lunch or supper?
- What would it be like if we had no one to care for us, or no friends?

Another way in which the topic could be introduced would be to consider the dependency of pets upon their owners – this would be particularly relevant if there happened to be a classroom pet. Many children have pets at home and a lively and informative discussion could be based on these children's knowledge of their pets.

The children could be invited to collect pictures, for a class wall chart, of all the things which help their pets to grow. A similar picture could relate to their own growth needs. Its form will clearly depend on their discussion but should include the four major components: food, exercise, rest and love and care.

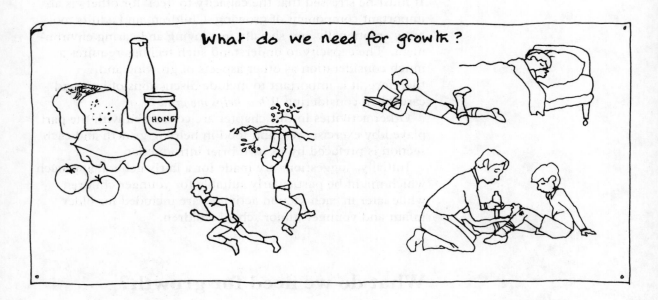

What do we need for growth?

Love and care

Someone caring helps me to grow

After a discussion, invite the children to make a picture of ways in which parents, directly and indirectly, care for their children.

Some ways in which our parents care for us
Going to work
Cooking food
Having fun
Taking trips and holidays
Looking after us when we are ill
Helping us grow
Washing our clothes
Making or buying our clothes

It is important that teachers, when discussing this subject, are sensitive to the different family backgrounds of the children in their class. The one-parent family, for example, is an ever increasing phenomenon in contemporary society and the teacher will need to approach this work with delicacy and a sympathetic manner. It may well be a good idea to stress the importance of 'adults', rather than use the word 'parents'. Most children will, of course, immediately think of their parents but it does mean that those children who have one parent, or who receive little love and care from their parents, will find it easier to identify with the example given. This matter is discussed further in the introduction to chapter 7 (*Knowing about others*).

In what ways do adults help us grow?

Ask children to describe a number of situations where they are cared for or helped by adults or parents. A story or a series of pictures might be used as a basis for such work:

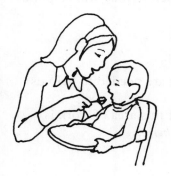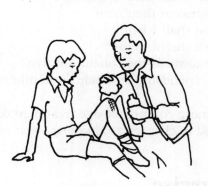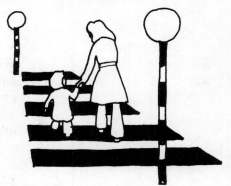

Ask them to think of a story to go with each picture.
– What could happen if adults didn't care for children?
– How do we learn from parents and other adults?
By watching, imitating and helping them, we learn to do things for ourselves.

Can we help ourselves to grow by helping others?

Part of growing is concerned with the realization that we do not need so much help and that we ourselves can offer help to others.

Ways we help others

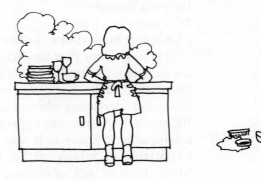

– How do I help?
– Am I helping my baby brother or sister to grow?

Ask the children to suggest ways in which each of them could help another person either at home or at school. They could write down, draw or dramatize these possibilities and discuss whether or not they could really be attempted.

After discussion, give the children time to put their ideas to the test – ensuring that they can be carried out simply and relatively quickly.

The teacher will probably need to offer several suggestions as to how children might help others before they will respond with ideas of their own.

– Who shall I help?
– How shall I help?

Work towards the conclusion that:

Love, friendship and help from others are needed to help us grow

 A more comprehensive treatment of this area of work is offered in chapter 7 (*Knowing about others*).

Exercise

The purpose of this section is to encourage children to participate in and enjoy a variety of physical activities. It must be remembered that these comprise both outdoor games and indoor activities such as movement to music, mime and drama, dancing, etc. The teacher may also wish to discuss with the children the function of bones and muscles and how they combine to allow movement of our limbs and other parts of the body. In addition, attention should be drawn to the place of rest and sleep in the cycle of human activity.

How we move

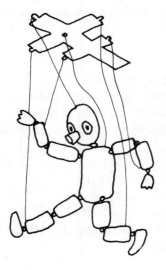

As an introduction to this topic, use a string puppet to demonstrate several different kinds of movement in its arms and legs. Ask the children to use their own bodies to copy these movements as closely as they can. Discuss with the children the similarities and differences between the puppet's movements and their own.
– What moves the puppet's arms and legs?
Ask the children to repeat their movements but this time to feel their muscles move (leg muscles are very noticeable on young children). Clenching a fist or waggling a foot will show results.
– What do muscles feel like?

Where are our muscles?

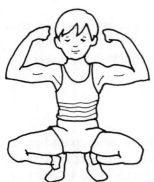

Ask the children to stand still and then to see how many different parts of the body they can move. Allow the children to explore their movements. Ask them to feel where they think their muscles are – this activity could be attempted during a 'movement' lesson. Discuss the reasons why we have muscles in most parts of our bodies.

Joints and Movement
Demonstrate again the movement of the puppet. Ask how many joints the children can see.
– What is a joint for?
  Ask the children to move about as if they did not have knee joints; to control a ball with stiff fingers; to lie on the ground and then get up with stiff (jointless) legs and arms.
  Try to bring into the classroom a skeleton, or, if this is not possible, some animal joints or bones.

What happens when I exercise?

Even young children could be asked to describe the changes which vigorous exercise brings to their bodies. Let them describe these changes in their own way after a suitable period of running or playing games.

– What words can we use?
– Can we make a song using these words?
– Can we make drawings to show what these words mean?

Older children might wish to consider, in a simple way, the reasons for these changes.

I feel hot because . . .

When muscles work hard they make extra heat.

The teacher might consider developing this area a little more by investigating with the children how excess heat is lost from the body – through the skin by evaporation of sweat.

I get out of breath because . . .

When muscles work hard they need extra oxygen.

Children might like to pursue the topic further by discussing what parts of the body are concerned with breathing, how the oxygen is carried to the muscles, and where it comes from in the first place.

My heart beats faster because . . .

It needs to pump more blood to carry the extra oxygen to our muscles.

Children could try to find out how much faster hearts beat after vigorous exercise.

How do muscles get stronger?

Ask the children how they think muscles develop and grow stronger. They could collect pictures of different sportsmen and sportswomen and discuss how athletes need to train in order to make their muscles even stronger, some developing

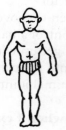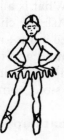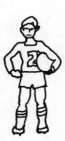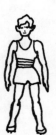

How do these people make their muscles strong?

52

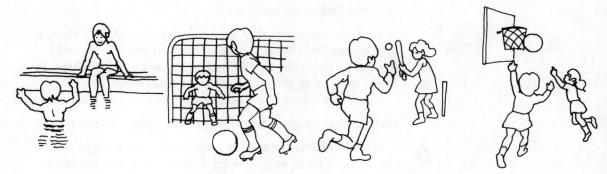

How do we make our muscles strong?

their muscles for speed, others for strength, control, endurance, balance, poise and so on.

Teachers might well include reference to the part played by food in making muscles strong and this is developed a little later in the chapter, on page 56.

Our favourite ways of taking exercise

Define exercise very loosely as those activities which use muscles a lot. Ask the children what they like to participate in and, if possible, encourage them to take part in some new activities.

Remind them of safe places to take exercise – playgrounds, parks, gardens, playstreets or other local facilities – and encourage, where practicable, the use of special clothing or at least *different* clothes.

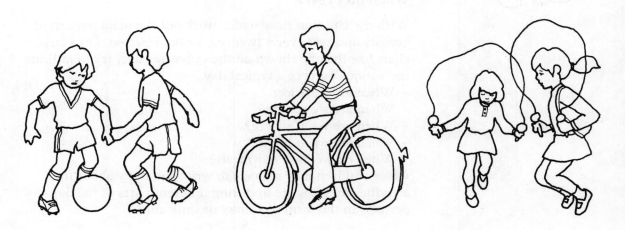

'Exercising' our feelings

It is most important that the children should have the opportunity to express their feelings in words, art and drama, so that they are helped to improve and perhaps to begin to control the expressions of emotions.

Ask them to use their bodies to mime words such as these:

very proud   angry   frightened   sad   shy   energetic   excited

Use situations to provide a reason for their expression of emotions. The strategies suggested in parts of chapter 1 (*Finding out about myself*) and most of chapter 7 (*Knowing about others*) could be of use here.

Rest

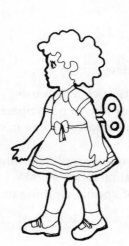

Why do we need rest?

In discussion with children develop the idea of the need for alternating periods of exercise and rest.

Allow children to watch a clockwork doll wind down, drawing attention to the slowing of its action until it stops. Ask how they are similar to and different from the clockwork doll.

The doll has a spring . . . the spring winds down.
We have muscles . . . our muscles get tired.
We can wind up springs but muscles need rest.

When do I rest?

With the children's assistance work out the main pattern of activity and rest over a twenty-four hour period. On a large chart like the one shown on the opposite page, try to indicate the various parts of a typical day.
- When are we asleep?
- When are we resting?
- When are we at school?
- When are we at home?
- When do we have our meals?

Older children may manage to write and draw about the activities they engage in during different parts of the day – perhaps in the form of a diary or timetable.

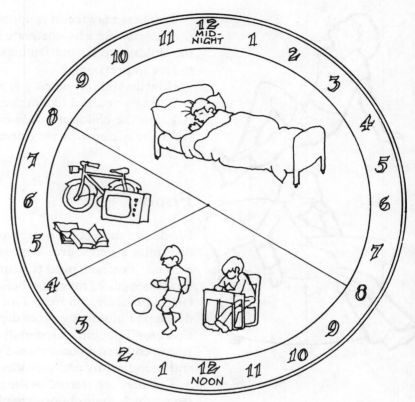

Why do we need so much sleep?

Before answering the questions directly, invite the children to find out about the sleeping habits of babies, themselves, and older brothers and sisters, discussing the relative needs of each.

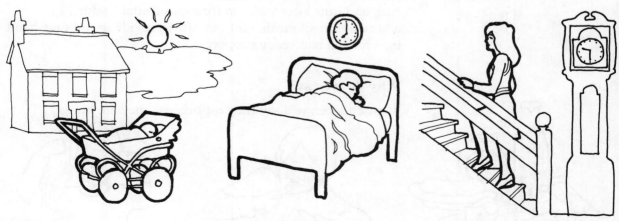

Babies need lots of sleep because they are growing so quickly

We need lots of sleep too, because we are still growing quickly

When we are older we will be able to go to bed later

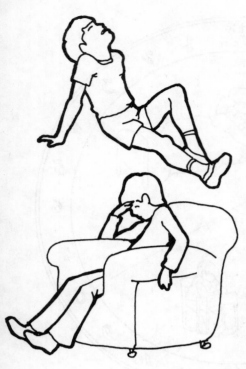

Teachers may feel it is appropriate to discuss bed times after discussing why adequate sleep is necessary. Arrange for the children to act out feelings of tiredness using their bodies to give impressions.

– How do you feel when you are tired?
– What do you feel like in the morning if you go to bed late? Ask how the children would explain to a younger brother or sister the reason why they need lots of sleep.

Food

Food, as a subject for topic work or as a centre of interest, does offer a rich source of possibilities for young children to explore. Teachers need to acquaint themselves with the fundamentals of nutrition before tackling this topic, particularly with older children. This subject is considered and developed in much greater depth in *Think Well* (unit 6, Food for Thought). Generally, however, it is sufficient for young children to understand that food helps them to grow and keep healthy and provides them with energy.

Teachers are alerted to the possible variety of backgrounds from which their children may come and, therefore, to the different kinds of food commonly eaten by them. It should also be remembered that families have widely differing food habits. Teachers might consider the use of school tuck shops, where they exist, to promote a sensible selection of snack foods. (Some schools have successfully introduced the sale of fruit and nuts after work on food and dental health.) In addition, school meals staff can often provide useful first-hand information and ready support.

Why do we eat?

Most children will say they eat because they are hungry.

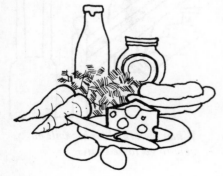
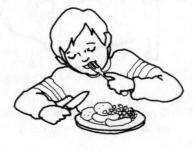
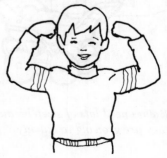

Without going into too much detail, relate the feelings of hunger to what the body needs for growth and energy. Remember that some children are very fussy about what they eat while others will eat almost anything. Eating for sheer enjoyment must not be ignored as a reason.

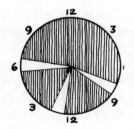

When do we eat?

Focus the children's attention on the pattern of eating times by looking at the times of particular meals. Draw attention to the different foodstuffs eaten at each meal. Remember that there will be great variation both in the times of the meals and the foods eaten at particular meals.

Which is the longest 'gap' between meals? Explain what breakfast means literally.

Why eat breakfast?
Point out how long the gap would be between the last meal in the evening and, say, school lunch, if no breakfast were eaten.
– How long does my 'fast' last?
– What do I have for breakfast?
Discuss the importance of starting off the day with a good breakfast.

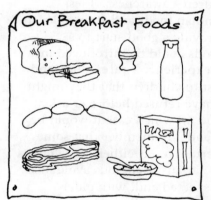

What foods do we like?

Using the pictures of 'Our breakfast foods' and adding others as appropriate, children can build up a wallchart of 'Foods we like'.

Invite the children to choose a meal they would like from the pictures displayed and, if appropriate, to draw and write briefly about the meal they have chosen. Teachers might also contribute a choice.

Display the favourite meals and discuss with the children the range of choices. This would be particularly relevant where the school has mixed ethnic groups.

It is important that teachers are not too critical of the 'favourite' foods; nevertheless it must be pointed out that eating too many cakes, biscuits, fats, etc, is not a good policy as these foods tend to lead both to dental decay and to fatness.

Is there a meal or dish which is particularly disliked by the children?

Trying new foods

Why do we like some foods and not others?

Ask the children to say which are their favourite foods.
- What do you particularly like about these foods?
- Is it what they look like, their smell, or their taste?

Ask the children to identify some foods by taste or smell only. Use this as a time for a safety reminder – don't taste unknown substances, etc. For further work on this topic see chapter 6 (*Keeping safe*).

Ask the children if there are any foods on the wall display of 'Foods we like' which they have not yet tried. Where there are immigrant children in the class, the number of foods that children have not yet tried is likely to be greater and this is an ideal opportunity to widen children's awareness of less common foods. For example, Indian foods and strange local names and specialities would provide a good start to a discussion. Perhaps different foods could be introduced into the display to widen children's experience – rarer fruits and vegetables, for example. Suggest to children that they might try a food at home which they have refused before or ask at home if they could try a new one (in which case it would be as well to warn parents beforehand!) Remember that some children will be unable to try certain foods either for religious reasons or because they are vegetarians. Religious avoidance of particular foods should be respected and, with older children, may provoke much interest and discussion.

Children 'experimenting' with new foods could be asked to write whether they liked them or not and why. A class record could be kept to encourage others to try the foods as opportunities are presented.

Children could make their own record by drawing a picture of the food, writing what kind of food it is and why they like or dislike it.

New foods to try		
Food	Experimenter	Result
Raw cabbage	John	
Leeks	Susie	
Liver	Pauline	
Curried egg	Margaret	

Jane's ... new food is ...cucumber

it belongs to the ...Fruit/veg... group

I tried it on Wednesday and liked it because

it was crisp and crunchy...

Food groups

With older children the teacher might wish to consider the topic of food in greater detail, in which case, as pointed out on page 56, the teacher should first acquaint herself with the fundamentals of nutrition.

One starting point is to make the distinction between foods from animals and foods from plants. Invite the children to make drawings or cut out pictures of foodstuffs which can be mounted on a wall chart under two main headings: 'animal' and 'plant'. Arrange the foods so as to allow for further categorization later and leave space for the addition of more cut-outs as work on the topic progresses.

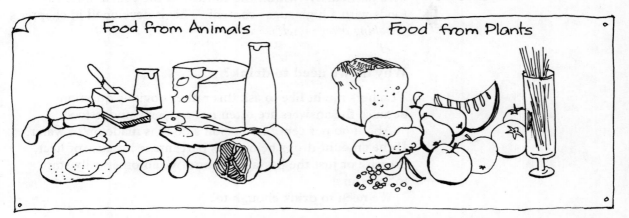

Explain that we need different kinds of food to help us grow, to give us energy and to keep us healthy. No one food does the job completely. There are three groups of food which are important to us and which are normally eaten every day. These three groups of food can be used to provide the children with a simple categorization of foods. This categorization will help children in food selection and will provide a sound basis for further work:

main part of the meal
fruit and vegetables
bread and cereal

With the children's help, rearrange the pictures into the above three categories. Teachers might wish to mention again at this point the fact that some people do not eat meat and are called *vegetarians*.

Building the wall chart could stimulate discussion not only about the placing of the foods but also about their origins.

Our Foods

Main part of the meal		Fruit and vegetables		Bread and cereal
Fish	Cheese	Brussel sprouts		Bread
Milk	Sausage	Potatoes	Peas	Various cereals
Bacon	Eggs	Cabbage	Beans	Cakes/biscuits
Chicken	Ham	Apples	Plums	Pasta

There are foods which do not fit neatly into these categories. What about butter, cream, sweets and chocolate? Do they make a real contribution to growth and good nutrition?

 The importance of food to dental health could be mentioned here particularly within the context of the consumption of foods with a high sugar content. This is developed in chapter 5 (*Looking after myself*).

Why do we need to drink?

Teachers might like to ask this rather obvious question because the answers are often not properly understood.

About 70 per cent of a person's body is made up of water. If the amount drops below this percentage because of heat, exercise or just the passage of time, we automatically start to feel thirst.

We need to drink enough to:

keep up the level of our body liquids (blood, saliva)
wash the waste and poisons out of our kidneys (urine)
help us perspire (sweat) so that we can regulate our body temperature.

It is often forgotten that food also contains water (nearly 78 per cent of meat and over 90 per cent of most green vegetables) and that half of the water we need we get from food.

We can survive for many days (even weeks) without food but only a very short time without water.

Ask the children to make a collection of pictures depicting the variety of drinks consumed by them.

– Do drinks contribute to our daily diet?
– What are they made from? What do they contain?
– Which is the most popular drink?
– Discuss the attraction of the most popular drinks and whether they contribute to the daily intake of food.

How food is prepared – keeping it clean

Many opportunities will present themselves for discussion of the need to keep food clean and free from germs. Work on hygiene and germs is dealt with in more detail in the following chapter (*Looking after myself*).

Discuss the different ways in which food is kept clean: wash hands and utensils carefully, cover food with a clean cloth, plastic film or put it into bags or airtight containers to protect it. Use boxes, tins, jars and the fridge.

Different ways of preparing foods
Discuss with children the different ways in which foods are prepared. Hold up a potato and an egg and ask them to think of the different ways in which each could be prepared.

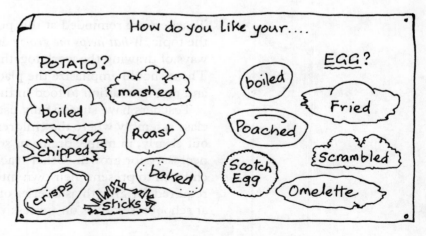

– Which method of preparation is the most popular?
– Which method of preparation is the least popular?

Children could be asked to think of how other foods might be prepared in different ways – for example, cheese, fish, cabbage, carrots.

If possible, have samples of the various methods of preparation to offer to children (particularly *raw* vegetables).

At this point teachers may wish to consider the importance of the 'milk' group of foods for growing children. Much useful work can be done by the children in making butter or cheese, or simply in learning that milk does not start life in the silver or gold topped bottle. (Suitable books, pamphlets, etc., are suggested in the Resources list, on page 125.)

Let's have a party

It would be appropriate, while this topic is being studied, to plan a class party or picnic which might coincide with a festival or holiday – harvest festival, Christmas, or suitable festivals related to other religions.

Discuss the variety of foodstuffs which could be brought by children and, if possible, plan to include some which would be new to children. Teachers will be aware of what each family could be asked to contribute so as to have a balance of food available. This could provide a useful and enjoyable conclusion to the work on food.

Concluding activities

Teachers are reminded at this point of the necessity to view the topic, *What helps me grow?* as a whole and to consider ways of drawing the work together in concluding activities. These should emphasize the place of love and care, exercise and rest in addition to food in the growth process.

Teachers have successfully used this topic as a focus for a class assembly where the children have been able to bring out clearly, in mime, drama or song each of the components necessary for growth. Other teachers have encouraged children to present their own interpretations of what is required for growth as a series of dramatized items presented at school assemblies on successive days of one week.

5 Looking after myself

Introduction

Young children can take pleasure and pride in doing things for themselves and this capacity should be harnessed in as many ways as possible. There are several areas of behaviour relating to health which lend themselves particularly well to the young child's desire for greater responsibility. Before looking at specific health practices, however, it might be of value to spend some time helping children to identify those areas of everyday behaviour in which they already help to look after themselves. This offers a 'centre of interest' unit for the early infant child and can be expanded where necessary to include more detailed discussion, information or instruction. We have examined in detail in this chapter three areas of health behaviour relevant to young children: dental health, hygiene and smoking.

The teacher has an important role to play in encouraging children to adopt favourable habits that will help to control gum diseases and dental decay. Both diseases start in childhood but can be prevented by careful tooth-cleaning and sensible restriction in sugar consumption. Established disease can be treated early so that toothache and unnecessary tooth loss is prevented. The responsibility for cleanliness, feeding habits and the use of health services lies primarily with the family. However, the teacher can provide a valuable link between the family and the dental profession and encourage children to be proud of their teeth and to look after them. Teachers might find it helpful to contact their local Area Dental Officer who may be able to arrange for talks on dental health or for children to visit a local dental clinic.

At first sight smoking might appear to be of little relevance to infant children. It is our firm conviction, however, that the attitudes of children towards the use of tobacco are already taking shape during the infant and early junior years of schooling. This is a time when they see parents, older brothers and sisters and perhaps even their own friends smoking, and they may therefore be motivated to experiment themselves.

Many children are encouraged by their social experiences to think of smoking as a 'normal' and 'natural' activity and which has little consequence for their health. In many subtle and more obvious ways they are also encouraged to associate smoking with physical toughness, attractiveness and many other desirable human attributes. We hope therefore that teachers will give consideration to the introduction of this area of work into the curricula of young children. Certainly the ideas related to smoking expressed in this chapter have been developed in many interesting ways by teachers who accepted the challenge to do something positive about the 'smoking problem'.

In what ways do I help to look after myself?

The following activities are primarily intended for younger children but are also most suitable for older infant children in terms of revising what they already know. Such teaching might usefully concentrate on the reasons why certain forms of behaviour are necessary or desirable.

The children will readily provide lists of actions they do during the day. One useful way of focussing this discussion would be to construct simple graphic diaries of the ways in which children help to look after themselves during 'My Day'. This might be compiled by the children individually in their own books or as a group or class activity. There will be many discussion points which can be expanded by the teacher as she feels necessary.

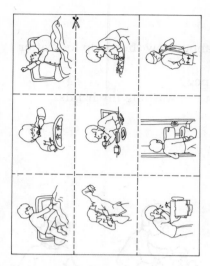

Spirit master sheet 5

My Day – At home in the morning

Sheet 5 of the *All About Me* spirit master book could be given to the children and they could be asked to cut up the sheet and then sort out the drawings into the correct sequence. Alternatively, the children's own drawings could be used.

Sorting out the sequence is of particular importance with regard to washing hands after using the toilet, a procedure which should be habitually emphasized and encouraged. With older children the questions should reflect their increasing responsibility:
– Do I actually get up when I am called? If not, why not?
– Can I find my clothes quickly in the morning?
Sheet 5 is also useful for work on the care of teeth, as described on page 68.

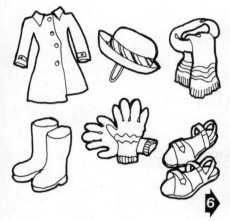

My Day – getting ready for school

– What do I need to wear?
– Do I need different things in winter and summer? Why?
– What do I need to take?
Pictures or word lists could be made of items such as dinner money, handkerchief, PE kit etc.

My Day – going to school

Discuss with the children briefly how they come to school – this will be covered in greater depth in chapter 6 (*Keeping safe*).
– Do I leave early enough?
– What do I do on the way?
– Am I ever late?

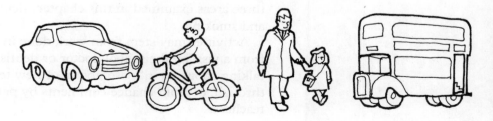

My Day – at school

Encourage the children to talk about how they help look after themselves at school:
- hanging up my coat – which peg?
- going to the lavatory . . . then . . . washing my hands.
- tidying up my desk/the toys . . .
- where do we put our rubbish?
- did I eat up my lunch?
- can I tie my shoe laces?

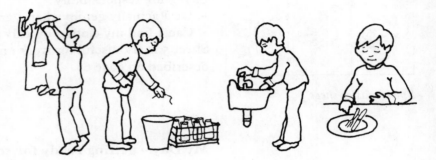

My Day – going home

- What should I wear?
- Who meets me?
- Do I cross a busy road?
- Do I go straight home?
- Strangers and me – what do I do?

My Day – at home in the evening

- Do I change my clothes/shoes?
- Do I brush my hair?
- What can I do to help?
- Do I clean my finger/toe nails?
- Do I go to bed when I'm told?

The general approach outlined above will provide starting points for a great deal of more detailed work, including the three areas examined in this chapter: dental health, hygiene and smoking.

Activities may stem from work done in preceding chapters, from a visit by the school doctor or dentist, from children talking about their 'loose' tooth, or new teeth coming through, or from chance comments by parents, children or teachers.

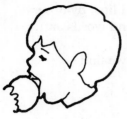
biting

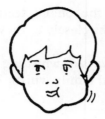
chewing

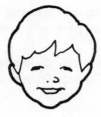
smiling

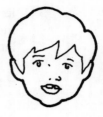
talking

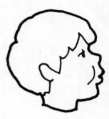
whistling

Looking after my teeth

What are teeth for?

A good and important reason for wanting to look after our teeth is that they enhance our general appearance – a fact which is not hard to impress on even young children.

Discuss the importance of teeth in smiling – study each other's smiles, collect 'smiling' pictures.
- Can we smile without showing our teeth? What happens? Ask a friend or look in a mirror.
- Can we look fierce by using our teeth?

A second important reason for wanting to look after our teeth is that they are necessary for biting and chewing food.

Look at bite marks in an apple or carrot. Try chewing a piece and describe the process.
- Why do we chew?
- Why must babies drink milk and eat soft food at first?

Either by studying a friend's teeth or by using a mirror encourage the children to observe:
- Which are our biting teeth? What do the others do?
- Our gums – where do the teeth start?
- How many teeth have you?
- Have you lost any recently?
- Are there any new ones coming through?

A third reason for looking after our teeth is that they are very necessary for clear speech. Children are often surprised to learn that teeth play an important part in the formation of sounds.

Certain consonants require the use of the tongue against the front teeth and some children with gaps in their first teeth will therefore have difficulty in sounding words containing these letters. Older children could attempt to discover which

letters make most use of the tongue, teeth and lips, by observing their partner's mouths closely as they sound words and letters.
— How many different ways of whistling can we find?
— Can all our friends and family whistle?

Wobbly teeth and what they mean

Children frequently need reassurance over two points concerning the loss of their baby teeth:

The loss of a baby tooth is usually the prelude to a new tooth appearing. The new tooth is already growing in the gums and will emerge when the roots of the baby tooth have dissolved.

The age at which teeth are lost and replaced is variable – some five-year-olds will already have lost some of their twenty baby teeth while others will have to wait until they are seven before this happens. Although the first permanent incisors replace the baby teeth, the first permanent molars come through behind all the baby teeth and do not follow the loss of any tooth. Many children and parents are thus unaware that a permanent tooth is now present at the back of the mouth. Children could be asked to look in each others mouths to see if the first permanent molars are there. Generally, however, the first permanent molars and the permanent incisors come through between six and seven years of age. The full set of thirty-two teeth is not complete until seventeen to twenty-one years of age.

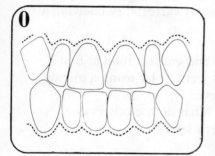

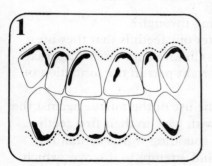

Cleaning my teeth

The primary aim of cleaning teeth is to remove plaque. Plaque is the thin film of bacteria (germs) which constantly builds up on teeth unless it is regularly cleaned off. Children can often scrape small amounts from their teeth with a finger nail. Another way of demonstrating its presence is by staining with a vegetable dye (such as cochineal). The plaque, which is normally whitish and difficult to see, becomes stained so that it now appears pink and is easily visible. One way of using a liquid dye is to put two small drops under the tongue and ask children to swish it around their mouths so that all the teeth are reached. An alternative method is to chew a disclosing tablet which contains dye. These are available at local chemists.

68

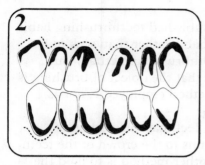

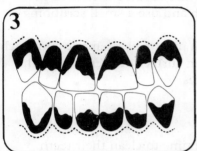

Teachers will find that children have varying amounts of plaque depending on their oral hygiene habits. Very few children will have no plaque. Some may have plaque covering a large part of the tooth surface. Teachers might like to score children on a scale from 0–3 depending on how much plaque is visible. Alternatively, encourage the children to carry this out for each other.

How can plaque be removed?
Older children might like to devise an experiment to find the most effective way of removing plaque. The class could divide into groups and try out different cleaning methods such as
– rinsing vigorously
– crunching an apple or carrot
– using a finger
– using a toothbrush
– using toothbrush and toothpaste
then stain the teeth with a disclosing agent and compare groups to see which method has been most effective.

Why do gums sometimes bleed?
It is difficult to actually damage the gums with a toothbrush, although very vigorous brushing with a very hard brush might harm the gums. However, children may notice that their gums bleed during the toothcleaning exercise. Healthy gums are a pale pink colour. Plaque irritates the gums and makes them inflamed. They become red and swollen and may bleed. Children should be reassured that it is not the brushing that is causing the bleeding, but the presence of plaque. If plaque is removed daily the inflammation should be reduced and the gums will no longer bleed.

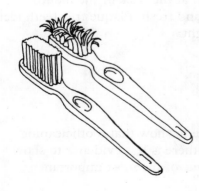

Toothbrushes
Children might be asked to bring their toothbrushes to school. A child's brush should be small enough to reach the back of the mouth (probably not longer than 1 inch, or even smaller for a younger child) and be renewed frequently. If the tufts are bent brushing cannot be effective.

When should brushing be done?
Plaque should be removed every day and children should be encouraged to brush after breakfast and before bed each night.

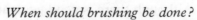

Methods of brushing

A child may already have an established toothbrushing habit. Teachers should build on that habit rather than seek to be dogmatic about one specific toothbrushing method. But always it should be emphasised that the object of brushing is to remove plaque. The exact method employed is not as important as the final result.

However, many dentists now feel that the method of sweeping the brush from the gums to the crown of the teeth is not particularly effective. Another method is to hold the brush at right angles to the teeth and use a small scrubbing movement.

Whatever method is chosen, it must be systematic and reach all corners of the mouth and each surface of every tooth, the inside, outside and biting surfaces.

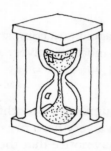

How long should brushing take?

It will take children much more time to clean their teeth effectively than most would normally spend. An eggtimer could be used to give a rough idea of the time that is required. It must be emphasised that we are aiming to remove all the plaque and this takes several minutes.

Help with brushing

Teachers might notice that children have very different abilities when brushing. Children who have difficulties with manual skills may also have difficulties with tooth cleaning. Young children may need help and teachers of five and six year olds might like to demonstrate by cleaning one child's teeth. It is helpful for the adult to sit or stand behind the child. This is also a useful time to point out how to reach the newly erupting permanent teeth at the back of the mouth.

A clean mouth feels healthy and fresh. Plaque free teeth feel smooth and look shiny and bright.

How sugar affects my teeth

Diet and Dental Decay

Although there is good evidence to show that toothcleaning can prevent gum inflammation there is less evidence to show that it prevents dental decay. One of the most important factors in dental decay is, in fact, sugar intake. It is important therefore that children are aware of the effect of sugar on their teeth. The idea that crisp foods such as apples or carrots are good for teeth is based on the misconception that these foods can effectively remove plaque. However, they are a suitable alternative to sugary snacks.

The frequency of sugar consumption
Most children are aware in some rather vague way that sweets are bad for teeth. However, generally there is less awareness of the widespread use of sugar in our society and the enormous amount that is consumed. In relation to dental health however, the important factor is not so much the amount which is consumed, as how often sugary foods and drinks are taken. Decay would be considerably reduced if sugar was limited to meal times only. Children should be encouraged to choose savoury snacks or unsweetened drinks between meals whenever possible. Teachers might consider realistic ways in which the school could influence children's eating habits. For example by attitudes to sweet eating in school, morning snacks, the sales in the school tuck shop and school meals.

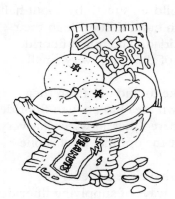

Spending pocket money
Many children have their own pocket money to spend. Teachers could discuss how much of this is spent on sweets. For example:
– when are the sweets bought?
– at school?
– on the way home from school?
– at the weekends?
– is the money spent on other sweet things such as sweet drinks?
– what alternative drinks and snacks are available?
– what fruits and vegetables do children like?
– do they like cheese and nuts?
– do they like milk?
– how many like water to drink?

How much sugar do we eat?
Children could collect food, drink and snack labels and look to see which contain sugar.
They might then try to plan food for a day with no sugar intake, with sugar on three occasions, i.e. at meal times only.

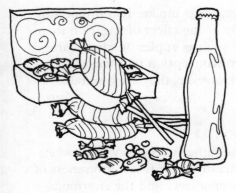

How can I limit the amount of sugar I eat?
- buy crisps instead of sweets after school
- bring cheese biscuits or an apple for lunch break
- spend pocket money on peanuts instead of chocolate
- drink water rather than sweetened drink when thirsty between meals
- have fruit or cheese instead of a pudding

Children might like to think up their own examples of how to cut down on the frequency of sugar intake.

Fluoride and Teeth

Have you got fluoridated water?
Carefully adjusted small amounts of fluoride in drinking water reduces the amount of decay in children's teeth by about half. A few local areas may have enough natural fluoride in their water, others may have fluoride added. Too much fluoride will cause a brown discolouration of the teeth, very small amounts will have no effect.

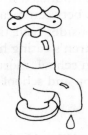

Teachers and children might like to find out from their local water board whether their own area has enough fluoride in the water. It should be remembered that all water has very small amounts of fluoride and that the optimal level is one part per million.

Most children in Britain do not have the benefits of fluoridated water. There are other ways of supplying fluoride although none are as good.

Other ways of getting fluoride
- ask the children to bring their toothpaste to school and find out how many contain fluoride
- have any of the children had fluoride painted on their teeth by the dentist
- do any children in the class take fluoride tablets

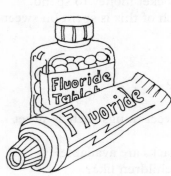

Visiting the Dentist
A visit to the dentist may be a considerable source of anxiety to children and even adults may be worried by the need for dental treatment. Indeed children's own fears may be learnt from adults conversation and for example the way that a teacher reacts to a child's request for absence for a dental visit.

Most children by the time they reach school age will have some experience of going to the dentist either for routine inspection or for fillings. Some will already have required the

72

extraction of a painful tooth. Teachers could discuss children's experiences. The positive benefits of early treatment and the relative ease of dental care with modern equipment and techniques could be explained to children.

Although the need for treatment is high in this age group many parents do not seek dental care for their children. School inspections are arranged for children annually and this is a chance for those who do not have regular care to be encouraged to attend the school dental service. Teachers could provide a valuable link between parents, children and dentists, and encourage early treatment when necessary, rather than waiting for toothache to occur.

The germs in my life

Children come to school with some habits of personal hygiene already fairly well established and these can be reinforced and further developed in school. Children's habits are more likely to be sustained if the reasons for them are made clear. Many starting points for this subject are possible: as a result of the work on teeth; children with coughs and colds; absences from school because of infectious diseases; local or national occurrences such as 'flu' epidemics.

The term 'germ' is used here to refer to a micro-organism (microbe) which is harmful to man. The size of germs is such as to make their description to young children a most difficult task and teachers are advised not to dwell too long on this concept. Teachers of older children are referred to *Think Well* (Unit 3, 'From Sickness to Health?') which considers wider aspects of the spread of diseases.

When asked by children specifically about size, however, teachers might usefully couch their answers in general terms as outlined below:

There are some living things in the world which are so small that we cannot see them even through a magnifying glass. These are called microbes. We need a very special sort of magnifying glass called a *microscope* to see them.

Not all microbes are harmful to man, indeed most are harmless. Some are even helpful, as are those required for the manufacture of cheese or yoghourt.

There are some microbes, however, that are harmful to man – these are called 'germs' and they cause colds, german measles, measles, scarlet fever and many other common illnesses. They are also responsible, as we have seen, for tooth decay.

Children should also be reassured that their bodies have very efficient ways of coping with germs but that they need to take some precautions nevertheless. Indeed, teachers should place the major emphasis upon what children can do to help protect themselves from the ill effects of germs. If people eat well, wash, rest and keep warm and dry, germs will be less likely to harm them.

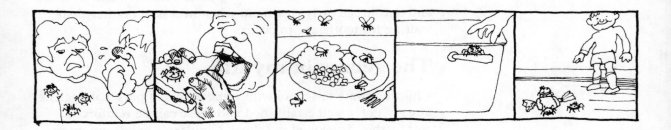

Ways in which germs spread

Discuss with children some of the more common ways in which germs are spread and ask them to illustrate by drawings, rhymes and drama how these might occur. Teachers might well start this work by supplying one or two ideas of their own.

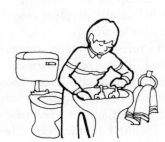

– sneezing and coughing at people and food.
– Handling food with unwashed hands.
– Flies from a dustbin landing on food.
– Not washing hands after using the toilet.
– Picking up and eating food from the floor.

Next discuss ways of reducing the spread of germs and invite the children to draw posters or make up rhymes about them:

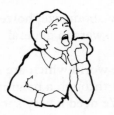

– Wash hands thoroughly with soap and water after using the toilet and before eating food.
– Use a handkerchief to 'catch' coughs and sneezes.

Teachers of young children have often found that songs, rhymes and simple role play are useful ways of stimulating interest in this work. For example, teachers could develop the following adaptation of *Simple Simon*:

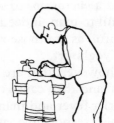

Simple Simon met the coldman going to the fair.
Said Simple Simon to the coldman, 'Who have you got there?'

74

'Its Coughing Sam,' the coldman said, 'Come closer if you
please, I'll tell you how we do our work, and spread lots of
disease.'

Children (or teachers!) could extend the rhyme to include
other suitable characters like 'Susie Sneeze', 'Fresh Air Fred'
and 'Eat Well Ed'. The rhyme could then be written and
illustrated, dramatized or made into a musical mime. Other
nursery rhymes, poems and songs could easily be adapted
in a similar way.

Stopping germs from making us ill – vaccination

It is important for children to understand that there are
other ways in which germs can be fought. They will no
doubt be familiar with the taking of medicines and possibly
also with vaccination. A fruitful and useful discussion could
emerge by asking questions based on a drawing such as the
one given on sheet 6 of the *All About Me* spirit master book.
- What's he doing? What does vaccination mean? Why is he
  doing it?
- Who has been vaccinated? What was it for? When? Where?

Some children may need reassurance that vaccination is
painless. Indeed, children may have the same kind of fears,
which teachers can do much to allay, about visits to the doctor
as they do about dentists.

Stopping germs from making us ill – medicine and pills

When introducing this topic two points must be stressed:

Medicines and pills are only used when we are ill.
They should be taken only when given by a doctor, parent or
nurse.
At all other times, DO NOT TOUCH must be the rule.

Ask the children to describe when they have had medicines
given to them. Use every possible opportunity to stress the
safety angle and to show that only parents, doctors and nurses
can know which is the correct medicine for an illness and how
often it should be taken. The children's descriptions could be
recorded to illustrate the process.

This might be a good place to explain that not all illness is
caused by germs and that medicines and pills are used to
treat pain or illness of many kinds. Most children will be

75

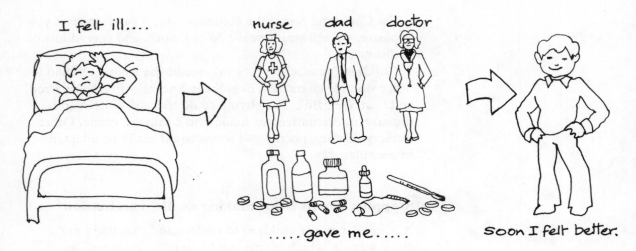

I felt ill....   nurse   dad   doctor   .....gave me.....   soon I felt better.

familiar with toothache caused by teeth cutting through gums and many will have been given small doses of aspirin to ease the pain. This might be a good example of a pain *not* caused by germs. Children could at this point be introduced to the idea of pain as a warning that something is wrong and may need attention.

 The work on the safety aspect of taking medicines provides a link with chapter 6 (*Keeping safe*). At this stage it is important that the children should recognize warning words such as:
CAUTION DANGER POISON
DO NOT TOUCH
KEEP OUT OF THE REACH OF CHILDREN
WARNING BY H.M. GOVERNMENT: SMOKING CAN DAMAGE YOUR HEALTH

Other ways I can help to look after myself and others

There are many other ways in which children help to look after themselves. Discussions and activities similar to those already suggested could be related to topics such as these:
My skin, nails and hair
My feet and shoes
My eyes and ears
For each topic children should think about: what they are responsible for and why; whether they should know how and

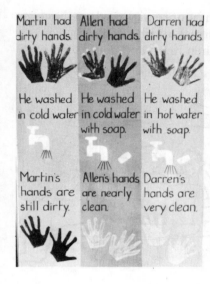

Martin had dirty hands. Allen had dirty hands. Darren had dirty hands.

He washed in cold water. He washed in cold water with soap. He washed in hot water with soap.

Martin's hands are still dirty. Allen's hands are nearly clean. Darren's hands are very clean.

when to carry out procedures; whether in fact they do what they know they ought to.

Older children might like to consider in more detail some of the topics suggested below, and present their findings to the class.

Helping skin do its work

- What does skin do?
- Why do we need to wash? (Dirt; grease; germs.)
- What happens if we don't wash? (Smell; itching; germs.)
- Where do we need to wash? (Face; neck; ears; under arms; feet; between legs.)
- When should we take special care? (Before meals; after using lavatory; after activity.)

Shoes and feet

How can we be sure they fit each other?
What are the sizes of feet and shoes in the class?

Do your shoes fit?
Draw round your shoe on a piece of paper.
Draw round your foot in a sock or tights.
Then draw round your bare foot or make a foot print.
How does your footprint compare with the size of your shoe?
Are your socks constricting your feet?

Further ideas are to be found in *Think Well* (unit 7, 'Get Clean').

Smoke and me

Whilst generally wishing to present the subject of health in a positive way to children, there are unfortunately several areas of health behaviour which can only be couched in negative terms, and tobacco smoking appears clearly under this heading. Nevertheless such work can be presented with humour, by using rhymes, songs or cartoons, for example.

Generally, however, teachers can usefully draw upon the experiences which children themselves have had at home and in other places.

Ask children to talk about their experiences involving

breathing in smoke – perhaps on bonfire night, when they have seen leaves and rubbish burned outside, when they are travelling in a bus or train, or when mum and dad have had a party in the house.

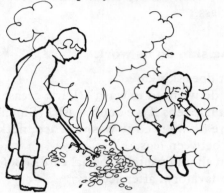 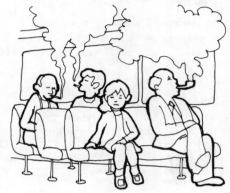

Has this ever happened to you?

– What do you think these children feel like?
– What effect do you think the smoke might have?
Ask the children to reflect for a moment and make a list of their comments, which might include:
– it makes me want to cough . . .
– it makes me want to choke . . .
– it catches in my throat . . .
– it makes me out of breath . . .
– it makes my eyes water . . .
– it makes my clothes smell . . .
– it makes me feel sick . . .
– it makes my throat tickle . . .

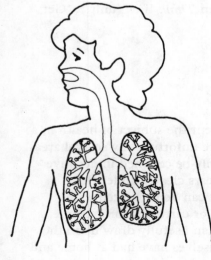

Invite the children to relate, write about or illustrate similar experiences which they might have had themselves:
– Where did it happen?
– When did it happen?
The teacher might wish to discuss briefly with older children why we need to breathe and how we do so, including the ways in which smoke can be harmful to the respiratory system.
– Why do we need to breathe?
– Which parts of my body are to do with breathing?
– What are they called?
– Why do we breathe faster after exercise?
– By how much does your chest expand when breathing in?
The work in this section provides a link with parts of chapter 4 (*What helps me grow?*).

Spirit master sheet 7

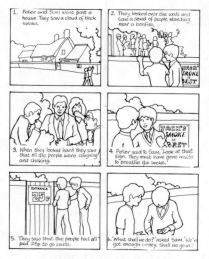

Spirit master sheet 8

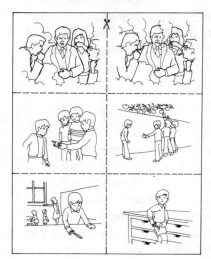

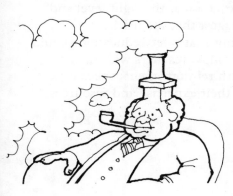

*If we were intended to breathe
smoke in and out wouldn't we
have been given a chimney in
our heads?*

The strange case of the Smoke Party

At this point teachers of lower junior children might wish to use the cartoon story shown on sheet 7 of the *All About Me* spirit master book. Read the story through with the children if necessary then let them draw their own conclusions and write or draw the sequel without further intervention. After they have finished it may be of value to discuss the picture sequence stage by stage using questions such as these:
– Do people normally stand in the smoke from a bonfire?
– There is a sign advertising smoke. Do people really try to sell it?
– What are the people doing? Why do they stay there?
– Lots of grown-ups have paid to buy smoke. Is it sensible then?
– They have all paid twenty-five pence. What for? To breathe in smoke?
– If you were the boys would you pay?

Teachers need to draw out conclusions from the story and also to make the connection between how both smoke from the bonfire and smoke from the cigarettes are harmful to our breathing system.
– Would Peter and Sam have been so interested if, instead of breathing in smoke from the bonfire, the people had been breathing in smoke from cigarettes or pipes?

Children could be asked to compare the illustrations shown at the top of sheet 8 of the *All About Me* spirit master book.
– Is there any real difference between breathing in smoke from a bonfire and smoke from a cigarette?

The children could extend their work by finding out what cigarettes are made of and by considering the ways in which the smoke from them is harmful to us. The work could well be concluded with a discussion about the 'advantages' and 'disadvantages' of smoking.

A full scale project on smoking (the Vectis Project) has been devised for older children and can be found in *Think Well* (Unit 4, 'Deadly Decisions').

6 Keeping safe

Introduction

Teaching about safety is important. In the context of health education one could say that if safety consciousness is not developed in a child then all other topics may well become irrelevant. Our aim is to provide children with the skills and awareness that they increasingly need on the roads, at home and elsewhere to keep them safe, without unnecessarily attacking their sense of adventure.

Safety education – whose job?

Teachers might consider that safety in all its aspects is the responsibility either of parents or of people with specialist knowledge such as policemen and Road Safety Officers, rather than themselves. The continuing large number of accidents to young children, however, indicates that the present level of preventive teaching is not enough. Moreover, teachers, unlike most other people, have both the skill and the opportunity for imparting information at the right level and at the right time. We do not suggest that the teacher supplants the efforts of others but that safety education should be the responsibility of many groups: teachers with their skills and authority; parents with reinforcement; specialists like Road Safety Officers, with their expertise and resources, in a supportive role.

How should we approach safety education?

Priority must be given to *training* children in safety measures. Making the subject interesting and enjoyable, for example with creative work, is important but must not obscure this primary purpose. The word training presupposes that safety education is not something to be tackled just once on a special occasion but rather that instruction is carried out regularly, for evidence suggests that the 'one-off' lesson achieves very little. It is important that the subject of safety should become part of a teacher's general approach.

Teachers should take advantage of any opportunities to make points about safety in different situations; during a walk or a visit; talking about homes; in the playground; going to and from school. In this way children should become safety conscious in a variety of different places and situations. This cannot, however, replace a structured school safety programme, where each class will cover matters appropriate to its needs and capabilities.

The approach to road safety

Infant children should not be on the roads by themselves at all. Research (as well as common sense) shows that, by and large, children of seven to eight years have abilities to cope with road situations that five to six-year-olds simply do not possess. Even these older children, however, have only limited skills: for example, they have difficulty both in judging the speed of a vehicle and predicting when it will arrive at a given point, and also in judging the relative speeds of overtaking cars. They also have problems in viewing traffic situations from other road users' points of view and thus predicting events.

The fact remains that large numbers of infant children do cross roads on their own. We therefore have an obligation to try. to develop their skills as far as possible and to help them to assimilate basic safety rules. As they grow older, children may begin to understand the reasons for these rules as they develop sufficient intellectual powers. There is no specific age at which this will happen, hence the need for continuous road safety teaching throughout this age-range. It has been found more effective to teach the younger ones 'a little and often' about road safety, whereas the older children may benefit from longer, more comprehensive lessons.

Another important point which has emerged from research in this field is that it is desirable and indeed necessary for *roadside* teaching of children to be included in a programme of road safety education. Teachers have often raised the problem of how best to organize visits to the roadside with small groups. Experience has shown that groups of ten provide a realistic number for such visits. Many schools have overcome the difficulty of providing sufficient staff for this roadside work by making use of teaching auxiliaries, parents, Road Safety Officers, students and other adults who are prepared to help.

A central part of a road safety programme should be roadside work on which other school work – such as model making, the designing of posters, charts, etc – can be based. Classroom activities are then seen to be related to the realities of local situations and have increased meaning and relevance for children. Similarly, visits to the school by road safety organizations and display teams should serve rather to supplement a structured teaching programme than to replace it.

Some schools have also successfully involved parents in their road safety work by telling them about what they were attempting and encouraging their active participation. Many parents have, as a result, extended such teaching into their homes where specific skills and vocabulary have been practised with their children. Such co-operation, while emphasizing the need to see safety education as going beyond the boundaries and influence of the school, nevertheless highlights the important part that teachers can play in the spread of safety education generally.

In this chapter, material on road safety is offered in three stages so as to correspond to the differing needs of children in the age group five to eight years. Teachers themselves are better able to relate such work to the capabilities of their own children but the three stages should be seen as a progression from the needs of early infant children through middle/top infants to the lower end of the junior school. No matter at what stage teachers decide to start their work, it is essential that all children are able to recognize and use the suggested vocabulary and it is recommended that teachers ensure that this is the case before proceeding to other aspects of the work.

Road safety: stage one

What do we know about roads?

Children need a sound knowledge and understanding of roadside terms. Questions using the appropriate words could be asked so that children learn to use them in the right context. The repeated use of the words is an important element of work with young children and for this reason teachers are encouraged to make simple games which match vocabulary with the appropriate pictures. A basic vocabulary might include the following words:

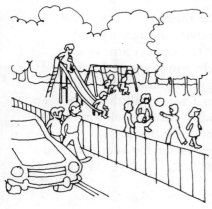

pavement   path road   kerb traffic
zebra crossing   pelican crossing   traffic island
car bus   lorry bicycle   motor-bike

It is important to emphasize the necessity of relating the vocabulary to the experience of the children; for example, in country districts where pelican crossings are extremely rare, this word might be omitted from the early work. The vocabulary could arise from early discussions with children concerning such questions as:

Where do we walk?
– Why don't we walk in the road?
Where do we play?
– Why shouldn't we play in the street?
Where do cars usually travel?
– Why don't they travel on the pavement?
– Are there some places where they do cross the pavement? (Driveways.)
Are there special places for people to cross the road?
– What are they called?
– How do we use them?

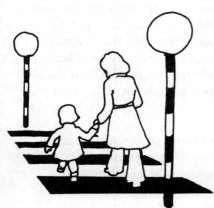

Discuss with the children why pedestrian crossings are safer. Remember to point out that they are *not* 'magic-carpets' and do not assume that children will already know how to use them properly.

A visit to the roadside

The earlier work can be consolidated and extended by a visit to a quiet roadside for a 'familiarization' walk. If the school is next to a road where the children can see traffic without leaving the school ground, this could be particularly useful.

Visits to the roadside are important for all children in order that they are better able to grasp clearly the ideas relevant to their safety on the roads.

Most children of this age find difficulty in combining different concepts. The points raised below regarding the sort of things using the road, the difference between moving and stationary vehicles and the idea of near and far, will all be fused together at a later stage. Children will then be able to make judgements about vehicle speeds and will be in a position to decide for themselves whether or not it is safe to cross the road.

What sort of things travel along our road?

This question is raised to ensure that children associate roads with large, moving objects. On their return to the classroom, children could make drawings and write the names of things that they saw travelling along the road. They could also make a collage or frieze of all the items seen.

Encourage the children to look for traffic in all directions – develop the idea that traffic might come from any direction. This will be a good foundation for later teaching concerning the Green Cross Code.

Moving vehicles

One of the skills that children need in order to cross the road is the ability to distinguish moving from stationary vehicles and to differentiate between vehicles 'coming' and 'going'. The visit could therefore provide an opportunity to practise this skill and to emphasize the fact that young children should not attempt to cross the road if they can see anything coming.

What is near and what is far?

Distance is a difficult concept for young children to grasp but could be practised with stationary objects at the roadside which could of course include parked vehicles. This could then be extended to include moving vehicles, although it should be stressed again that young children should not cross the road if they can see anything coming.

Which things on the road are most dangerous to us?

Children usually associate speed and danger with large vehicles such as buses and lorries. The teacher could point

Spirit master sheet 9

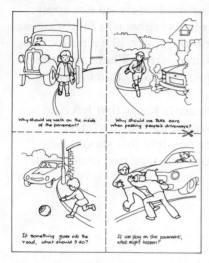

Spirit master sheet 10

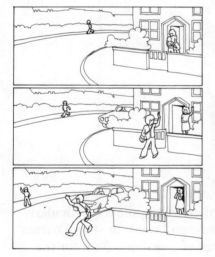

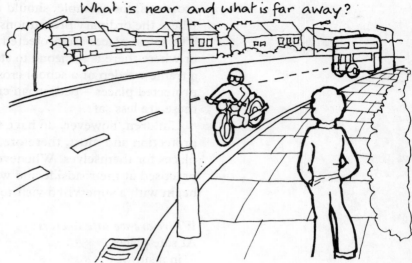

What is near and what is far away?

out that cars and motor cycles go fast too and are just as dangerous, and that bicycles are small and very quiet.

What could cause an accident?

Arising out of the previous work or, better still, following from a second roadside visit or walk during which teacher and children look for possible danger spots in their own environment, the children could discuss possible dangers to themselves as pedestrians.

Children could be shown illustrations of situations such as those shown on sheet 9 of the *All About Me* spirit master book. The question 'When might we forget to look?' could usefully be asked with some of these situations. (Children frequently say they did not see the car that hit them.) The children could make up pictures of their own for these situations. They could also be given for discussion a picture story sequence such as the one shown on sheet 10 of the spirit master book.

Road safety: stage two

Where is it safe to cross?

The first part of the Green Cross Code says, 'Find a safe place to cross then stop'. The word 'safe' worries several road safety experts. They are anxious that zebra and pelican crossings, for example, should not be seen as 'magic carpets' where the ordinary precautions of road safety do not apply. The safest places are protected places: subways; footbridges; or where there is someone to stop the traffic like a policeman, a traffic warden or a school crossing patrol. There are other protected places – pedestrian crossing and traffic lights – but these are less safe.

Children, however, do have to cross roads that have no protection and must, therefore, learn to find the safest places for themselves. Whenever possible this should be practised at the roadside and work on stage two could well begin with a supervised visit to a busy road.

Where are we safe to cross?
At safe places:
   in a subway
   on a footbridge
   on a zebra crossing
   on a pelican crossing
With safe people:
   with a policeman
   with a lollipop man/lady
   with a traffic warden
   with an adult we know

– Why are these places safer?
– Why must we still take care?
– What must we look for?
– What must we listen for?
– What must we do?

Stress the need to take care at crossing points (particularly zebras) since the traffic needs time and room to stop. Discuss the special requirements of types of crossings. Wait for the cars to stop, the signal to be given, walk straight across still looking and listening.

Invite the children to compile 'sets' related to:
- things that move fast on the roads
- people and things that help us to cross roads safely

Make friezes of:
- Safe places to play
- Safe places to cross a busy road

each of these should depict local situations known to the children.

86

Who helps us to cross the road?

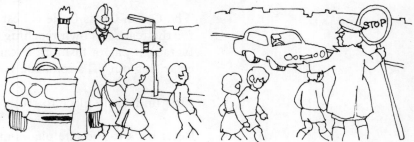

Children often like to draw pictures or write about people who help them. Visits and talks from people like policemen or lollipop men can be useful, but *only* if they know how to talk to small children.

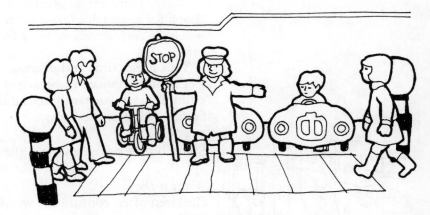

Some schools have children role-playing crossing the road. Maximum use can be made of this by insisting on the right procedures such as stopping before crossing, waiting for a signal and so on.

Crossing the road

There is no real substitute for the actual practice of crossing the road in small, supervised groups, although it can be useful, when at the roadside, to talk about where and when to cross. In tests with children it has been shown that even though they know the 'right' answers to road safety questions their behaviour on the road is more often than not quite different. To develop understanding of this complex code needs both training and practical experience, there is no other way.

The Green Cross Code

The Green Cross Code is best viewed as a sound framework for the teacher's own teaching programme and ought not to be taught parrot fashion. It can best be introduced during, or arising out of, a roadside visit.

1   First find a safe place to cross, then stop

Refer back to the safe places mentioned in the earlier work. Lower juniors will need to be taught to distinguish the safe from the unsafe. One way to begin this might be to use pictures like the ones shown on sheet 10 or sheet 11 of the *All About Me* spirit master book to stimulate discussion.

Where there are *no* protected places children should: 'Look for a stretch of road where you can see *clearly and far enough in each direction*, away from road junctions and parked cars.'

This needs time and practice.

The importance of *stopping* at the kerb needs stressing to children who constantly see adults step straight off the kerb, looking as they cross.

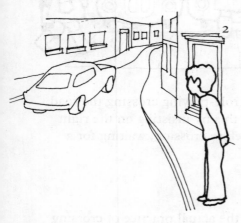

2   Stand on the pavement near the kerb

What is the kerb?
Children often confuse the words 'kerb' and 'curve'. Point out how to recognize the kerbstone and what it is for.

Where is 'near' the kerb?
Children think of this as anything from standing with their toes over the edge to one metre back. A distance of 15–20 cm from the edge is recommended and this should be demonstrated.

The emphasis is on being able to see clearly while being safe.

3   Look all around for traffic and listen

The instruction, 'look all around' has sometimes resulted in children rotating their heads but seeing very little. Alternatively, they often interpret it widely and look in front gardens or at the sky. They should be encouraged to concentrate on specific details relevant to their crossing, identifying what they see and hear. Stress the following aspects:

Things which are on the road and moving
Children have difficulty in distinguishing between parked and moving vehicles in the distance. If things appear to be moving they should not cross.

All the places that traffic could come from
Remember both directions, round a corner, close in to the kerb, parked. Bicycles seem to have a habit of appearing silently from 'nowhere'.

The traffic noises that they can recognize
One school recorded different vehicles slowing down, speeding up and braking to make a training game for the children to identify certain typical traffic sounds.

4   If traffic is coming let it pass. Look all around again

Emphasize here being patient and continuing to look in different directions until there is no traffic near.

5   When there is no traffic near, walk straight across the road

Discuss what 'near' means in this situation. Again remember that young children cannot judge speeds, overtaking or arrival times.

YOUNG CHILDREN SHOULD NOT CROSS IF **ANYTHING** IS COMING

Why straight across? Why not at an angle?
The children could try both ways in the playground and could count how many steps they take. If the distance is greater, will it take longer to cross? Stress that 'straight across' is the shortest and therefore quickest way to cross the road safely.

6   Keep looking and listening while you cross

Children need to be given plenty of opportunities to think about the operation of the Green Cross Code and to act out

89

its meaning for them. Teachers can offer such opportunities in many different ways:

- Actual road crossing situation under supervision
- Simulated road crossing situation in school playground using children on bicycles, etc, as traffic.
- Using pictures or photographs or a child crossing a road successfully using the Green Cross Code.
- Having 'older' children teach the code to others in the class.
- Having children think of a 'play' in which the Green Cross Code is featured.
- Constructing a game based upon 'snakes and ladders' in which during a journey to school the ladders are represented by successful completion of one of the codes (from the Green Cross Code) and the snakes are represented as violations of one of the codes. Dice or other means of random choosing numbers might be used as in 'snakes and ladders'.

It is emphasized once more, however, that the concepts basic to the Green Cross Code need to be reinforced by work throughout the early life of children and should not be seen as a once-and-for-all effort or the part of schools or teachers.

Road safety: stage three

Coming to school

It would be fruitful now if children were to identify the kinds of hazards and dangers which they individually meet on their way to school. The individual safety requirements of children can be clarified by finding out which method they use to come to school. Children themselves could produce a block graph to illustrate this.

How do we come to school?
- How many children walk to school?
- How many children come to school by bus?
- How many children come to school by car?
- How many children come to school by taxi?

Children could be encouraged to describe, in writing and drawings, the safety measures they each might take in response to the possible hazards met on their way to school. This might be developed as, 'My personal safety plan' or, 'My personal guide to safety' and incorporate many of the ideas from the previous two stages.

How we come to school																	
I come to school on my own																	
I come to school with a grown up																	
I come to school with an older brother or sister	1	2	3	4	5	6	7	8	9	10	11	12	13	14	15		

I COME TO SCHOOL BY CAR
- Where should I sit?
- Do I have a safety harness?
- Where do I wait?

Liaison with parents could be most useful here. It should be emphasized that children ought to *sit* in the *back* of the car, never in the front unless it is absolutely necessary, since adult seat belts never suit small children.

I COME TO SCHOOL BY BUS
- Where do I wait for the bus?
- Do I have to cross any roads to reach the bus stop?
- How do I wait? Am I standing too close to the kerb?
- Are there rules for getting on the bus?
- Are there rules for getting off the bus?

I WALK TO SCHOOL
- Do I cross any roads? Are they busy or quiet?
- Are there zebra crossings I can use?
- Is there any other kind of help to cross busy roads?
- Do I walk on my own?

This may be a good point at which to raise the idea of not accepting help from strangers, only people that they know are safe.

Coming to school in bad weather or when it is dark
If this kind of observation can be done in the actual weather conditions or at night, so much the better. With a view to practicalities, however, it might be better if, over a period of time, a teacher could build up a series of slides of the same local traffic intersections in a variety of weather conditions. Questions could then be based on these illustrations:

When it is *raining* . . . when there are *leaves* on the road . . . when there is *snow* on the road . . . when it is *icy* . . .
- Can cars stop quickly?

– What might happen if they tried?
– What might happen if they skidded?

We must take extra care when roads are slippery
When it is foggy or dark . . .
– Can we see easily?
– Can drivers see us?
– How can we see cars or bicycles?
They put on lights
– How can they see us better?
We put on light-coloured clothing

We must take extra care when it is dark
This would also be a good time to introduce the idea that vehicles cannot stop immediately.

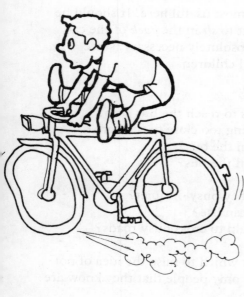

Can cars and lorries stop straight away?
It is obvious to adults that vehicles cannot stop 'dead', but it will need explaining to children. One possible way to illustrate this is to tell them to watch at traffic lights or pedestrian crossings where vehicles have to stop. Do they just stop or do they have to slow down first?

Children could easily prove this to themselves by using their own bicycles and tricycles. If they ride them across the playground and put their brakes on at a certain chalk mark, they could then measure how far they travelled before they stopped. The connection with motor vehicles should then be made.

The construction of a model or map of the area surrounding the school could also draw the attention of children to the purpose of road signs and traffic lights. It would be opportune to discuss with older children the colours that are used for traffic lights.

What are traffic lights for?
– What colours are the lights? What do they mean?
– Which colour signals danger?
– Which colour signals 'free to go'?

Our area

It is very important that children are able to recognize and to see at first hand their own local hazards. Generalizations are insufficient – teachers need to specify where hazards are present in the locality. To this end teachers often compile sets of photographs or slides emphasizing 'safe' crossing points, basing these photographs on work done with children in their own locality.

Models and Maps
Older children could trace a local map to show their route to school. They should mark features such as their house, school and crossing places. They could then identify danger points and work out the safest route to avoid them.

It is often helpful for children to identify the best place to cross by a feature such as a pillarbox, a particular shop, or 'the white gates'.

Many schools make models of the roads in their area, putting in buildings, road signs, crossings and other local features. These models can prove extremely useful for demonstrating situations that could occur on the roads in the area. The relevance of road signs nearby can be discussed, and the use of toy figures and vehicles could usefully pose several questions such as:
– What traffic is on the road?
– Are there any dangerous places?
– Can this man see those cars round the corner?
– Which are the safest places to cross the road?

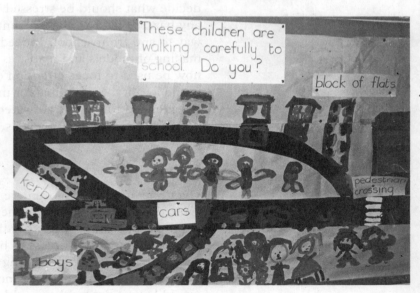

Such work will enable the teacher to focus particular attention on the dangers presented by crossroads or bends.

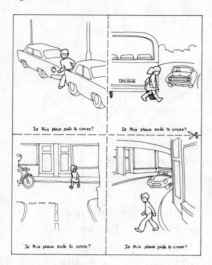

Illustrations like the ones shown on sheet 11 of the spirit master book would be a good starting point.

Discuss with the children the dangers of crossing the road at crossroads or on a bend. Can they think of a safer place? There is ample opportunity here for the children to write about the things they have seen and to draw their own examples of dangerous places they know. The abler ones may be capable of using the situations as a basis for creative writing.

Keeping safe outside

The kind of work that can be done in school with regard to outside safety is much less sharply defined. There may be some dangers to children outside their own or other people's houses: pesticides in sheds, garden tools, machinery, etc. Dangers of this kind can, however, be drawn into discussions on home safety.

Other dangers may be particular to an area: tips, demolition sites, abandoned houses and cars, canals and rivers, for example. We think it best left to the individual teacher who, on the basis of knowledge of her children and locality, can decide what should be stressed. She should consider especially any hazards likely to be encountered by the children on their way to and from school. Indeed, it is suggested that the making of models and maps (as outlined on page 93) should now be used to focus attention on other danger spots specific to the locality. Such a map or model could, for example, be extended to include all water hazards in the neighbourhood – rivers, streams, pools, canals, etc.

Swimming

Over one hundred children are drowned ever year in the United Kingdom, therefore the importance of teaching children to swim properly hardly needs emphasizing. Many schools do now have access to baths where children of this age can have regular swimming lessons.

If swimming instruction is not available at the school it would help if the teacher could point out to children and parents the days and times when classes are available to them at the local swimming baths.

Keeping safe at home and at school

Much of the work suggested for this section is concerned with the recognition and avoidance of danger. It is clearly beyond the power of children of this age to actually change a dangerous situation in the home. It may be, however, that with parent/teacher co-operation, a home safety campaign could be organized which would involve hazardous situations being recognized and remedied. Indeed several schools have successfully involved parents in such schemes. The object should be to show children how accidents can happen, but to avoid frightening them and to keep a constant emphasis on prevention.

Infant and lower junior school teachers are of necessity safety conscious and will be aware of the dangers particular to their school and classroom – swinging doors, low windows, difficult stairs, etc. We have therefore kept suggestions about school safety to a minimum and concentrated on the home where far more accidents occur.

Have many accidents ever happened to us?
This provides an interesting opportunity to focus the attention of children on accidents generally.
– Has anyone fallen down?
– Has anyone burned themselves?
– Has anyone fallen off a bike?
– Have we had any accidents in school?
– How did they happen?

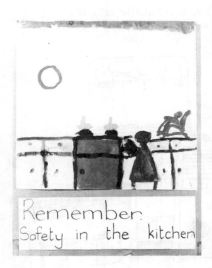

Remember.
Safety in the kitchen

Could we have stopped them happening?
It is important that the sensible way to avoid each accident should be an important part of the discussion. One school made a 'dangerous-sounds' tape accompanied by pictures of the items recorded, such as:

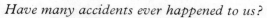

fire crackling	bottle breaking
kettle boiling	power drill
door slamming	lawn mower

Discuss with the children how some of the accidents already noted could have been prevented. Invite them to make simple 'posters' for use at home and school and which cover some of the important points raised.
● Clear away toys – this prevents other people tripping over them.

- Never leave any object on the stairs – this can be particularly dangerous.
- Be helpful by keeping your eye on younger brothers and sisters.

This section is linked strongly with chapter 1 (*Finding out about myself*) and chapter 7 (*Knowing about others*) in its accent upon personal responsibility.

Do we have any safety rules in our school?
This might well arise following questions about accidents in school. In one school a book of safety rules was produced, written and illustrated by the children themselves. This will also present a good opportunity to revise the 'fire drill' adopted by the school.

Taking care indoors

Fires, burns and scalds
Almost every school has its share of 'latch-key' children many of whom are frequently at risk from the articles shown in the illustration below.

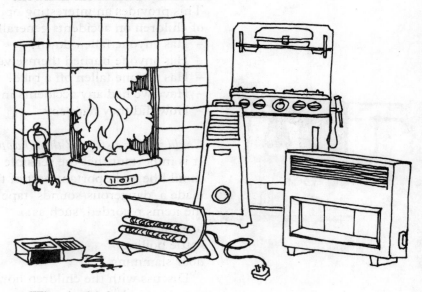

- What is this?
- What is it for?
- Have we got one?
- Is it dangerous?
- Can we make sure it won't harm us?

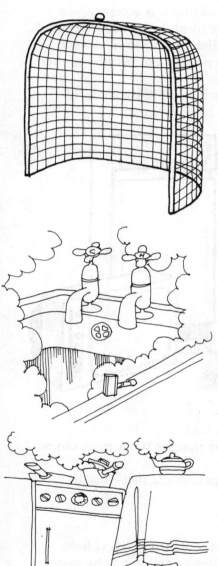

A classroom display of articles or appliances which could be dangerous to young children could be used to stimulate discussion. Discuss simple safety measures for each item. It would be particularly useful if the actual articles could be brought into the classroom for teacher and children to examine and discuss.

Older children could conduct a class survey of the kinds of heating and cooking appliances used by their parents and also of the rooms in which they are likely to be situated. Many children have produced drawings of homes, based upon the survey, illustrating the kinds of heating and cooking appliances available and these have provided a focus for much written work, discussion and role playing. For example, where homes have open fires the use of a fireguard provides an interesting stimulus to discussions and drama.

– What is this for?
– How does it help to keep us safe?
– Have we got one at home?

NEVER PLAY NEAR A FIRE

Teachers might wish to consider with children ways in which 'fire precautions' or even a 'fire drill' would be appropriate to their own home. They could draw up a poster or pamphlet for their own homes covering points such as:

WHAT SHOULD I DO IF A FIRE STARTS?
Warn others as quickly as you can.
Ring the Fire Brigade, night or day.

GET OUT AS QUICKLY AND CALMLY AS POSSIBLE

Make sure parents or other adults call the Fire Brigade however small the fire seems.
If you remember to, close doors on the way out.

– How many ways can I get out of the house if there is a fire?
– Can I use a telephone? Do I know how to ring for help: fire, police, ambulance?

The dangers of hoax calls could well be discussed with junior children.

It is helpful also to identify specific rooms where burns or scalds could occur.

Children could usefully be asked questions about illustrations like those shown on the left.

– What can you see that is dangerous? What can be done about it?
– What are these for?
– When do we have them?

- Who can buy them?
- Who looks after them?
- Who lights them on Guy Fawkes night?
- Do you know the firework safety code?

NEVER PLAY WITH FIREWORKS

Electricity – friend or foe

The use of electricity is so general that it is accepted as a normal part of life – yet it can be most dangerous if misused in any way. Children are particularly prone to its dangers because of their ignorance of its powers and because of their innate curiosity.

Children could build up collections of illustrations of household appliances that work by electricity.

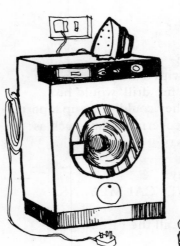
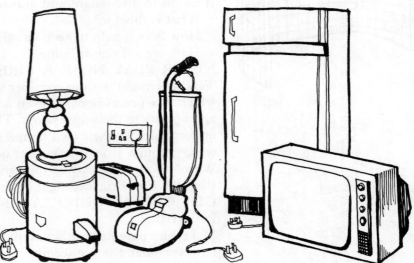

- Could these be dangerous? Why?
- What are the wires and plugs for?
- Should we plug in and unplug things? What parts can we touch?
- Draw pictures of all the things at home that work by electricity.

Poisons and Medicines

One of the most successful ways in which teachers have approached this subject with younger children is by using 'safe' and 'unsafe' tables. The safe one is covered with green and the unsafe with red. A variety of foods, containers and bottles are collected by the teacher, and the children tell her

onto which table she should put each item. Onto the safe table would go food, drinks, sweets and chocolates. Onto the unsafe table should go anything the children consider dangerous, or are unsure of. Examples are shown in the drawing below. Use *pictures* of different coloured pills especially those that look like *Smarties* or jelly beans.
ALL CONTAINERS SHOULD BE CLEANED AND RENDERED SAFE BY THE TEACHER BEFORE BEING BROUGHT INTO SCHOOL

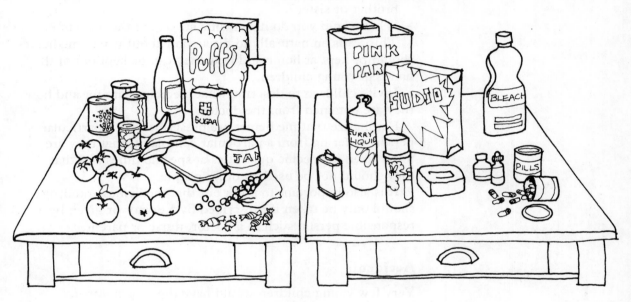

- What is this?
- What is it used for? If you don't know, *don't touch*.
- Is it dangerous? Why?
- Where should it be kept?

Very important additions are bottles that do not contain the original liquid, such as a *Ribena* or squash bottle with a different liquid inside (water will do for a demonstration).

- Do we know what is inside this bottle?
- Is it safe to drink? Is the label always right?
- What should we do if we find a bottle like this?

Sweets and Pills
As a development of this work, some teachers have filled and sealed several bottles with sweets resembling pills of different kinds and colours while having other carefully sealed bottles filled with pills. The children have been invited then to guess which are sweets and which are pills. This has led to

99

interesting and important discussions resulting in children acting out situations where strange 'sweets' have been found by young children:

at home

in the street

in a train

in a bus

- Can you tell the difference between sweets and pills?
- What would you do if you were looking after a younger brother or sister?
- What would you do if someone ate one of the 'sweets'?

This leads on naturally to discussion about where medicines should be kept at home and how they can be kept out of the hands of young children.

Invite children to describe what medicines are for and how they are obtained from the doctor.

Emphasize that medicines are prescribed for a particular person suffering from a particular complaint, that they are to be taken in specific quantities at specific times and that they should not be used by other people.

It is also important to point out that medicines and drugs should only be taken if prescribed by a doctor or given by a responsible person such as a doctor, nurse or parent.

Accidents

Very few young children would have the capacity to act thoughtfully after an accident. They can, however, be taught some skills and procedures that are useful now and may well be developed as they grow older. This would also be a good time to emphasize the importance of the telephone as a means of communication which could result in the saving of life. For this reason it is a means of communication which should not be abused by acts of vandalism or by indulging in hoax calls.

- Do you know your name, address and telephone number?
- If there was an accident at home, who would you tell?
- If mum and dad weren't there, who would you tell?
- Could you use the telephone to call for help?

Discuss how to use it and what they would need to say. Older children should be able to manage an emergency call from a call-box.

- If you haven't got a telephone at home do you know where the nearest call-box is?

– Can you make a telephone call from a call-box?

The emphasis in any discussion, written work or drama should be upon contacting the most suitable adult as rapidly as possible.

First aid

The first duty of infant and lower junior children in any emergency should be to get help as soon as possible. Infant school children are obviously too young for a detailed course in first aid but can be encouraged to do helpful things in an emergency as outlined in the previous activities. There is however a Junior Red Cross Safety Course including elements of first aid and this is aimed at the eight to eleven years age group. Further details of the course can be obtained from the local British Red Cross Association.

It is suggested, however, that teachers should acquaint themselves with at least the rudiments of first aid procedure and local authorities frequently provide courses for this.

7 Knowing about others

Introduction

As discussed and emphasized in earlier chapters, children in their early years have already begun to build images of themselves as a result of their relationships with others – particularly with others of importance to them. An additional and important part of the social development of children is concerned with learning to live with others, making friends, learning about their society and its values and beginning to understand about some of the rules by which we all live.

The family, of course, plays the major role in the early social development of children, for it is in the family situation that the foundations of learning to live with others are laid. Through identifying with and imitating parents or other adults who are important to them, children adopt attitudes, values and perspectives which markedly influence the way in which they relate to others. Thus, being able to have respect for others, to feel love and compassion, to develop the capacity to share, take turns and offer help are, essentially, human traits which are, in most cases, initially nurtured within the family.

While recognizing the importance of early family experiences we must remind ourselves that the process of socialization does not cease at any particular point. It is a dynamic process which continues throughout the life span but which does retain at its core many early experiences to which constant reference is made. New situations are met and handled by recalling past experiences where similar problems were dealt with, successfully or otherwise. The social experiments of school life are important adjuncts to and developments of such early socialization, and can offer many new opportunities for the young child to add to his core of experience.

The school is a community which offers to children opportunities for social interaction which will almost certainly be of a different kind or quality to those found at home. It is a community where sharing, helping, taking turns, understanding and obeying simple rules may take on a new importance. For the first time children meet with experiences not readily available elsewhere: experiences which spring from involvement with many other, often very different, children. Learning about others and the range of behaviour which falls into the category of 'acceptable' and 'normal' is an important part of learning to live with other people.

We have concerned ourselves in this chapter with three important groups within which children's early social experiences will take place: the school, friends and the family. Within each we have developed the concepts of belonging, sharing, helping, taking turns and understanding about rules.

We begin by looking at school as it is one area of experience which will be common to all, and which provides ideas and strategies which teachers themselves can develop. We realize that some teachers will, naturally, be a little apprehensive about tackling such work and we would like to offer a general reassurance, based upon the experiences of teachers who have worked through the strategies with their own classes, that such fears are unfounded. Teachers reported improvements in relationships between children and generally appreciated the sharpened awareness they themselves developed of individual children in their classes. Anxieties seem to have disappeared as a result of becoming involved in activities which teachers saw as contributing to the development of children as social beings.

Our section on friends is an extension of the concepts of belonging, sharing, etc, into the narrower and special world of 'us' as a small group, sharing common experiences. The topic of friends will probably have more relevance to the seven- to eight-year-old than to the five- or six-year-old.

A section about the family has also been included for the simple reason that families are important to children and will provide some common ground for discussion. Teachers become particularly anxious when they are considering topics which appear to intrude upon the family life of children and for this reason this area of work is developed at the end of the chapter after they and their children have had an opportunity of becoming better acquainted. Teachers must, however, consider seriously the implications of dealing with this area, and may need to examine their own assumptions and expectations concerning what the 'family' is. Families can be one-parent families, two-parent families or may be extended to include grandparents or other relatives. Often the family includes a widowed grandparent or uncle or aunt who might play the role of 'mother'. Families can also have other extensions – the child may have two 'mums': his 'proper' mum and another 'mum' who his dad may have married. Similarly some children may have two 'dads'. The teacher setting out to study the family must be sensitive to the range of expectations and understandings which children will bring to this work.

Many teachers will doubtless ask, 'Can we really help children to develop insight into their own feelings and those of other people?'

There is no simple answer to this question but if one believes that 'learning to live with others' is indeed an important part of the process of education, then there is but one answer: an emphatic 'Yes'. Perhaps we might rephrase the question to read, 'How can we help children to develop insight into their feelings and those of other people?' The rest of this chapter gives teachers some suggestions for work with the children which may help to answer this question to their own satisfaction.

Finally, although much of this work does lend itself to written and other work of a more tangible kind, much also is dependent upon discussion, drama and role playing – work which is less easy to record and display. The latter type of work however is no less important in the development in children of an understanding which contributes to social awareness and responsibility.

Together in school

What makes the classroom ours?

The following ideas are suitable for work with younger

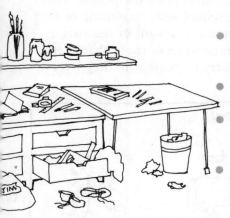

children. Discuss with them how they know that the classroom belongs to them.

● What is 'mine' and what is 'ours'.

| my teacher | my peg | my table | my tray | my picture |
| our teacher | our pegs | our table | our trays | our pictures |

● I share the classroom with other children – what else do we share?

● The things we do make the classroom ours.
   – Why do we need to keep the classroom tidy?
   – Whose responsibility is it to keep the classroom tidy?

● We all belong to the class. We all share in the classroom. To belong we must make a contribution – we must help.

How can I help to keep the classroom tidy?
   – In what ways do I help to keep the classroom tidy?

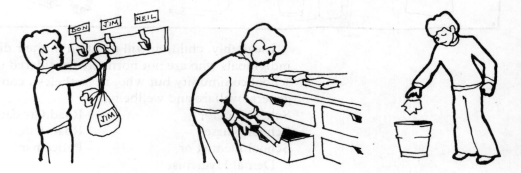

Who helps us in school?

The work in this section is more appropriate for older children and many teachers have developed the theme into a main topic or project centred on the school community. Its major purpose is to direct children's attention towards those people who contribute to their welfare. Children are often surprised to learn of the different kinds of services provided for their benefit by various individuals, and such a project can offer a basis for understanding the interdependence of members of the community.

Discuss the school as a community and the need for sharing the kinds of jobs which have to be done in schools amongst a number of people.

Find out whether the children know the names and titles of the people who help in the school.

Invite some of these people to talk to the class, but first ensure that they are used to talking to young children. The

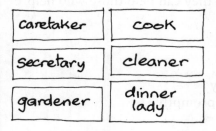

caretaker	cook
secretary	cleaner
gardener	dinner lady

– *In what ways do these people help?*

class could make a montage of pictures of all the people who contribute to the running of the school and, by writing or in discussion, describe how each person plays his or her part.

Children could be asked to mime some of these characters in front of the class which could try to guess who they were supposed to be.

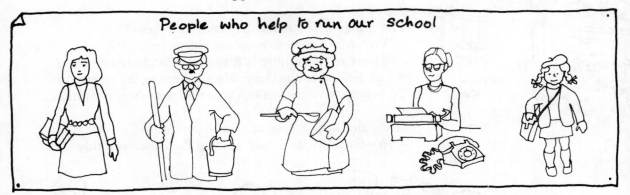

People who help to run our school

Inevitably, children will mention in their discussions individuals who are not normally considered to be part of the school community but who, nevertheless, contribute to its general welfare and wellbeing.

School Doctor
School Nurse
School Dentist or
  Dental Hygienist

Road Crossing Officer
Road Safety Officer
Policeman

There are obvious connections here with the work of other chapters, particularly with chapter 5 (*Looking after myself*) and chapter 6 (*Keeping safe*).

Children need to be reminded from time to time that they also have responsibilities and should not consider themselves merely as recipients of the services of other people.

How can I help?
Discuss with the children how they can help those who help them.
By picking up litter
By keeping things tidy
By being polite
By remembering dinner money
By returning letters and notes promptly
By obeying instructions
By taking notice of 'rules' if any.
– Are there other ways of helping those who help us?

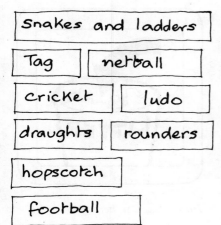

Are there rules for us to obey?

It would be appropriate first of all to discuss with the children the purpose and function of 'rules' in different kinds of situations. We do not wish to convey an impression that rules should be obeyed unthinkingly or mechanically but rather that they should be considered in the light of what they were intended for.

Ask the children to think of games they play which have rules. Discuss with them what they think rules are for.
- Why do these games need rules?
- What would happen if they didn't have rules?
- What will happen if we don't stick to the rules?

What are our school rules?

If there are any school rules, this would be an opportune time to discuss with the children what they are and the reasons for them. Teachers should be prepared for challenging questions on this topic, particularly from older children.

Most rules are made to help people or to protect them or their property

Invite each child to imagine himself as someone who has to make and uphold rules for other people. Then ask the children to explain who they are and the reasons for their rules. The teacher might have to allocate roles to the children. Some examples are:

I am a park keeper
I am a librarian
I am a teacher

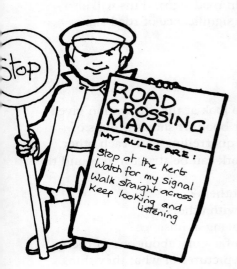

Do we always obey the rules?
- Do we understand them?
- Do we forget what they are?
- Are we too lazy to obey them?
- Perhaps we don't care about others?

There are obvious connections to be made here with chapter 6 (*Keeping safe*). It would make sense to consider some rules for safety at home, at school and on the road. This may include a discussion of road signs.
- What signs can we make to remind us of some of the rules for safety at home or at school?
- What about other rules?
- What might happen if we ignore them?

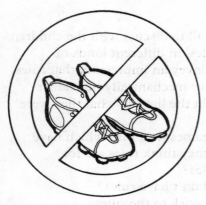

Orders – must be obeyed.

Warnings – of possible danger.

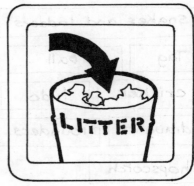

Information to help.

Older children might be encouraged to make signs based upon the code of shapes used in road signs. This will also sharpen their awareness of the significance of road signs generally.

Do we help each other?

The children could be asked to look at the illustration given on sheet 12 of the spirit master book. It shows groups of children, helping, sharing and quarrelling with each other. Much language and written work can be structured round this picture.
– Which children are helping others?
– Which children are sharing with others?
– Are there children who are being a nuisance?

Invite the children to think of a story about one of these situations and to write or draw pictures of what they think would happen next.

Spirit master sheet 12

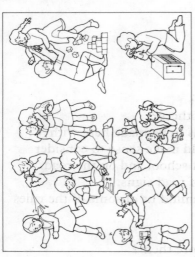

Do we quarrel with each other?
Inevitably, the teacher often has to mediate between children who are, for one reason or another, at odds with each other. Frequently such occasions can be used as starting points for discussion about quarrelling. Teachers can, alternatively, use a sequence of pictures such as those shown on sheet 13 of the *All About Me* spirit master book. These will focus attention on such a problem.
– Why are the two boys quarrelling?
– Have you ever felt like either of these boys?

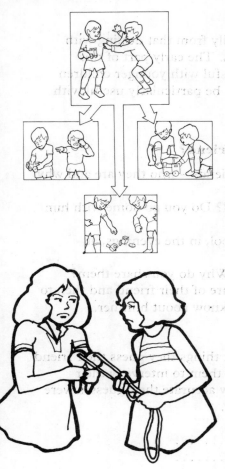

Spirit master sheet 13

– What happened in the end?
– What do you think will happen next?
– Look at the three ways in which this quarrel is likely to end and decide which you would like best if you were one of the children.
– Why do you think the boy is crying?
– In what ways have these boys decided to end their quarrel?
– What do you think these boys are feeling?
– Are there other ways in which the quarrel might have ended?

If there is sufficient interest, perhaps the children could start a *How to stop a quarrel Book* which could relate instances of how quarrels begin at school and outside. Invite the children not only to describe the quarrel itself, but also to make suggestions about how it could have been avoided or resolved in a way that would please those concerned.

– Why are these children quarrelling?
– What do they feel like?
– How could they end the quarrel happily?
– Does this kind of thing happen often?
– What could they do?

Sometimes quarrels start when we are playing games and someone doesn't know or obey the rules, or as a result of teasing, calling each other names, or merely not wanting to join in.

Our Co-operative Plan

Some teachers of older children have found it useful to introduce the idea of a group or class plan in which the children will need to co-operate in determining and achieving their goals. Class plans need to be prominently displayed in order that all members of the class can see what the aims are and what their individual contribution is to be. A few suggestions are offered:

- picking up litter – why, where, when?
- doing a play or assembly – about what, who, how?
- doing a collection of wool or silver paper for . . .
- constructing a plan of the classroom – who does what?
- making models or pictures as a group – of what?
- decorating the classroom – with what, from where, how?
- making group/class booklets – what size, shape, colour, contents?

My friends

This section follows on naturally from that dealing with school and school relationships. The early part of this section has proved very successful with younger children while the latter part is likely to be particularly useful with older children.

What do I know about my friend?

Ask the children about their friends – who they are and why they are 'friends'?
- Do you live near your friend? Do you go home with him/her?
- Do you play together at school, in the evenings, at weekends?
- What things do you share? Why do you share them?

Ask children to make a picture of their friend and then to write or draw everything they know about him/her.

I guess my friend would like
Children might be asked to list things they guess their friend would like. After guessing, ask them to interview their friends in order to find out how accurate their guesses were and what they have missed out.
My friend likes
(T.V. programmes) . . . .
(food) . . . .
(pets) . . . .
(comic or book) . . . .
(pop star) . . . .
(sports personality) . . . .

Keeping friends
Young children are of course constantly changing their friendships and there is no implicit assumption here that children must or 'should' form lasting attachments with others, although this often occurs. Nevertheless it would be useful for children to look in a simple way at the kind of behaviour which they generally accept as being desirable in friends.

Using a strategy similar to that in chapter 1 (*Finding out about myself*), allow children to play out roles in front of the others and discuss with them the sorts of personalities more likely to retain friendships.

Teachers might use for discussion characters from stories or books familiar to the children.

Cheerful	Charlie	or	Cheryl
Happy	Hamil	or	Heidi
Fierce	Ferdinand	or	Felicity
Jealous	John	or	Jean
Quarrelsome	Kenny	or	Karen
Noisy	Nick	or	Nisar
Argumentative	Andy	or	Alison

– What kind of person would you be friendly with?

Why is my friend my friend?

This might be a very difficult question to answer as children will tend to answer, 'Because I like him/her', using the word 'like' to mean a multitude of qualities. However, their awareness can be increased by looking for several different dimensions of friendship, although this activity is more likely to appeal to older children.

– we live near each other
– we enjoy doing things together
– we both belong to Sunday School
– we go to Cubs/Brownies together
– he/she shares toys with me
– he/she is kind to me
– he/she is cheerful and good fun
– he/she is always happy

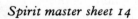

Spirit master sheet 14

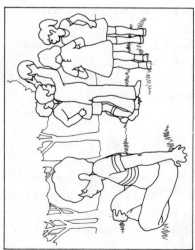

What are friends for?

Ask the children to look at the picture on sheet 14 of the *All About Me* spirit master book and to describe the scene. Invite the children to comment on the behaviour of the boy which could have led to the situation. Afterwards, discuss whether he could do anything to help the situation or whether the members of the group could. Try these questions:

– Does the boy want to be on his own, do you think? Why then, is he alone?
– Is there anything the boy could do if he wanted to join the group?
– If you were a member of the group what would you do?
– What would happen next? Finish the story off in words and pictures.

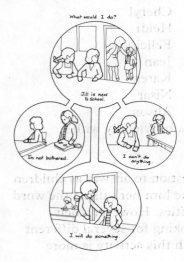

– If the boy was new to school today, how could you help him feel better?
– Has this ever happened to you? What did you do? How did you feel?

Making friends 'What would I do?'
Children often find themselves in new situations where they have no friends or acquaintances. A typical situation occurs when a new child comes to school and is ignored by the children in the class.

This sequence of pictures shown on sheet 15 of the *All About Me* spirit master book is provided for teachers to broach such a situation with the children.
– How do you think the 'new girl' feels on her first day at school? Are there any words which might describe this feeling? Have you ever felt like that?
– What do you think the girl in the bottom picture is saying to the 'new girl'?
– Why do you think the other girls are acting the way they are?

Follow my leader

The purpose of this section is to develop in children a critical awareness of behaviour. It would be appropriate for junior children.

Discuss whether it is always good to be one of a group. Ask children if they can think of situations when people prefer to be alone, or to do things on their own. Discussion may be made easier if the children are encouraged to write their thoughts down first.

Things I like to do alone	*Things I like to do with friends*
I like to	I like to . . . .
. . . . on my own	. . . . with my friends
because	because . . . .
	. . . .

Do I always do what my friends do? What should I do?
Ask children to look at the illustrations shown on sheet 8 of the *All About Me* spirit master book (shown on page 77).
– Would you accept the cigarette? Would you take apples too?
– If you do not act like the group, what may happen?
Discuss the 'dares' which children sometimes give each

other and how some of them can be dangerous not only to themselves but also to others.

If my friend does something wrong . . .

Invite children to comment on an open-ended story such as the example shown on sheet 8 of the spirit master book.
– How did this situation arise?
– How might it end?
– What would you do if this was your best friend?

Spirit master sheet 16

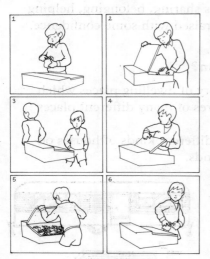

What are the things you could do?
– Ask why your friend had taken it.
– Ask him to put it back.
– Threaten to tell teacher.
– Tell teacher – Tell his parents.
– Do nothing.
– Which is the *best* for your friend?

This situation was deliberately structured to provide no possible ambiguity. Many incidences of 'stealing' are not so clear cut since the objects taken and motivations differ from case to case. While in no way condoning stealing, teachers have a duty to explore the background to such situations and to look for possible explanations. Another incident involving stealing of property belonging to someone else is illustrated on sheet 16 of the *All About Me* spirit master book. Again it would be interesting to explore with the children some of the possible reasons for such a theft.

What reasons might there be for a boy to steal the sweets?
– Might he not have enough money to buy some for himself?
– Would this excuse the theft?
– Is he just greedy?

Am I made to want things?
Older children can also begin to look at how the media influences their behaviour – particularly in increasing their range of 'wants'. Some teachers have helped their children to develop interesting and sometimes humorous topics along the following lines:
    Collect adverts of all kinds aimed at children – for toys, comics, sweets, clothes, etc.
– What makes me want things?

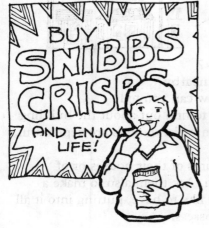

– Who puts ideas into my head?

Make adverts for: 'How to keep friends' and 'How to get into the school team'.

Homes and families

Teachers must remain alert to the fact that 'home' can encompass a wide variety of situations and that children will bring with them to school many different kinds of experience reflecting their interpretations of home life. Teachers should, therefore, introduce this topic with some delicacy. There are, however, common ideas such as sharing, belonging, helping and taking turns which can be raised with some confidence.

What places do people live in?

Discuss with children the variety of dwelling places which are used as homes. Make pictures of many different places where people live.

Ask the children to look for different kinds of houses on their way to school or at weekends.

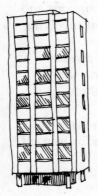
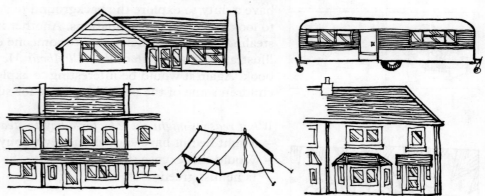

– Are they new or older houses?
– Are there houses being built nearby?
– If so, what sort are they? How can you tell?

Older children have gone on to find out about the building materials used, different ways in which houses are kept warm, and so on.

Invite children to make pictures of their houses or of homes they would like to live in. Ask them also to make a picture of the room they would like to have, putting into it all the things they would like to possess.

Teachers have been surprised by the wealth of detail which some, mainly older, children have put into their pictures including such details as the kind of heating used, how the house might be insulated, details of gardens, etc.

What is a home for?
The teacher might wish to discuss with the children, in very simple terms, what a home is for.

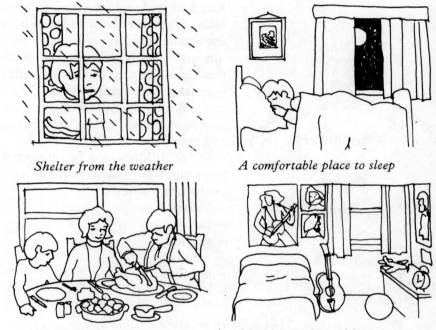

Shelter from the weather

A comfortable place to sleep

A place for the family to eat

My place to keep things

- What are the kinds of things we do at home?
- What can we do to make our home safe?
- In which rooms do we need to be particularly careful?
  Clear links can be made here with chapter 6 (*Keeping safe*),
- particularly those sections relating to keeping safe at home.

My home and family

Ask each child to think about his home and the people who share it with him. The children could draw pictures of and describe their family members, or alternatively, could bring photographs, including those of their pets, to stick into their books.
- Who lives in my home?
- Who shares my room?

- Who looks after me?
- Have I any pets?
- Where are they kept?
- Who looks after them?

What is a family?
Discuss what the children understand by the word 'family'.
As was mentioned in the introduction to this chapter, there
may be a wide range of responses here. It is important that
each child feels that his idea of a family is equally valid and
the teacher should particularly encourage children with more
'unusual' family backgrounds to respond at this point. If the
teacher is not careful, 'family' will be synonymous with two-
parent nuclear family. Whatever form the family takes, it
remains a family in that it is a fairly permanent group of
people and it serves the basic needs for love, care, protection
and training.

Older children may be interested to see how wide apart
(geographically) their 'families' can be while still maintaining
contact as a unit.
- loving
- caring
- sharing
- helping
- teaching
- learning

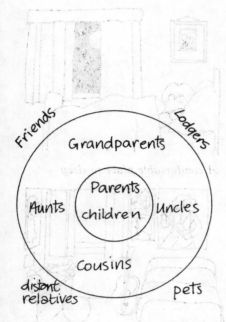

How do we come to belong to a family?
Teachers might wish to discuss how some individuals are
born into a family, while others are adopted by a family.
The important point to stress when this topic is being discussed is that whether we are born into or adopted by a
family, we are wanted and are an important part of it.

How do we know that we belong to a family?
Family names and what they may mean could provide
interesting discussions, particularly if there are immigrant
children in the class.
- When do we change our names?
- What was my mother's name before she married?
- How many different last names are there in my family?
Where we live indicates membership of a family group, and
so does *Knowing that we have relatives* and keeping in touch
with them.

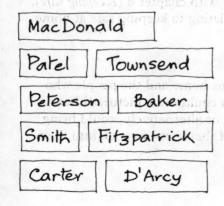

Ask the children to record in words and pictures how their families keep in touch with each other by:

Visits
Phone calls
Letters
Photographs

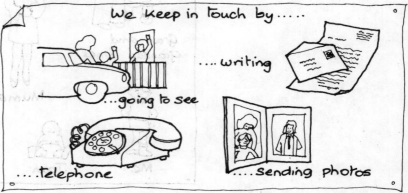

Encourage the children to write a letter and send it, with some drawings, to a relative or a friend of the family whom they have not seen for some time. Older children could bring in letters from relatives and, by studying the postmarks and addresses, mark on maps where they have come from.

This has proved to be a successful idea with older children and has served as a useful introduction to larger spatial concepts. One relative, a member of a crew of a merchant ship, wrote to his nephew (and the class) from each port of call and the children traded his progress on a large map of the world which they had constructed themselves.

Do families come together? When does this happen?
Invite children to make a picture of 'My family get-together for . . .'

Holidays	Weddings
Christmas or other religious festivals	Christenings
	When someone is ill
Parties	Funerals

Where do we belong in our family?
Junior children might be capable of, and enjoy, constructing a simple family tree. Ask them, concentrating on the family members that are close to them, to make a family tree starting with the oldest first.

– Who is the oldest in your family?
– Who is your oldest sister or brother?

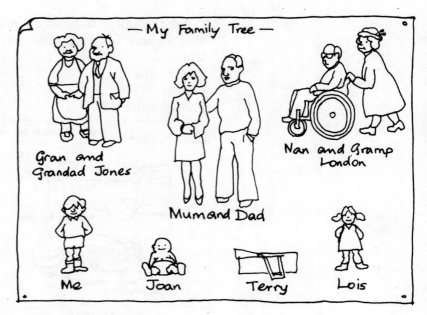

— My Family Tree —

Gran and Grandad Jones

Mum and Dad

Nan and Gramp London

Me

Joan

Terry

Lois

- Who is the youngest?
- Is it better to be young or old?
- Is it better to be a boy or girl?

Sharing with the family

Ask children to compile pictures of the kinds of things families do together.

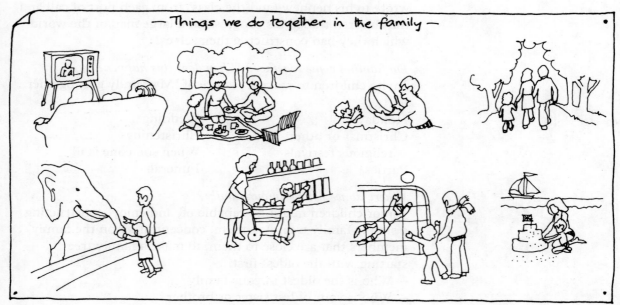

— Things we do together in the family —

What else do we share in the family?
Often certain 'shared' family possessions are sources of
potential and real conflict between family members. Such
common possessions could be television sets, radios, record
or cassette players, pets, books, games or games equipment.

Interesting discussions could follow on from role-playing.
Pairs of children could act out situations where two members
of a family have conflicting aims, desires, etc. Children can
be invited to adopt roles by 'wearing other people's glasses',
'stepping into someone else's shoes', 'wearing someone
else's hat' or by wearing the appropriate clothes.

Teachers of younger children are often presented with such
opportunities when children are allowed to dress up and
imitate adults. Similarly Wendy House play can offer
situations of potential conflict which can be used to advantage
by the teacher to illustrate the need to consider the feelings
of others.

Wearing other People's Glasses
This idea is best used with children of junior school age.

The teacher should have ready several pairs of spectacles
without lenses, or cardboard replicas, each clearly labelled
with the name of a family member – gran, grandad, mother,
older sister, older brother, etc. When children put on these
glasses, they must try to behave as that named person. The
spectacles can be used in many different kinds of family (or
other) situation to stimulate interesting, and at times
humorous, discussion. Try to introduce the children to
situations which occur fairly frequently in the family such as:
– Who chooses the television programme?
– Is it too noisy? (Playing the radio, record player, etc)
– Who cleans out the pets?
– Whose turn is it next?

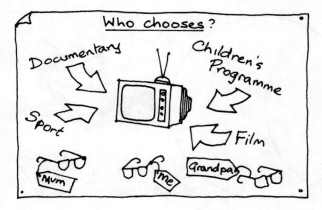

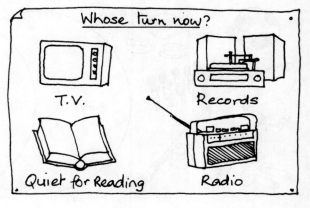

Allow the children sufficient time to think about their roles. Help them to think out how such people would feel about the situation and how they would react by asking questions such as the following:

— What would he/she think and say?
— How would he/she act?

Further ideas are developed in *Think Well* (Unit 1, 'My Self', and Unit 2, 'One of Many').

Does it matter whether you are a boy or a girl?

Teachers might wish to consider how male and female roles can be reinforced by the jobs boys and girls are asked to do, the games they are expected to play, etc. It would be enlightening to discover how far children have already determined their sex roles. It may well be found that there are differences in the degree to which this has happened which will produce different responses to the activities suggested below. Discussion centred on these activities, and in particular on any variations of response, could be used by the teacher as a good starting point from which the children can be encouraged to question the traditional sex roles.
At this point, if there are any school jobs that are always done by children of one sex, the teacher could change the system to one where all jobs are done by children of both sexes.

— What are some favourite girls' activities?
— What are some favourite boys' activities?
— What are some activities which both boys and girls like?
— What are some jobs that boys do?
— What are some jobs that girls do?
— What are some jobs that boys and girls do?

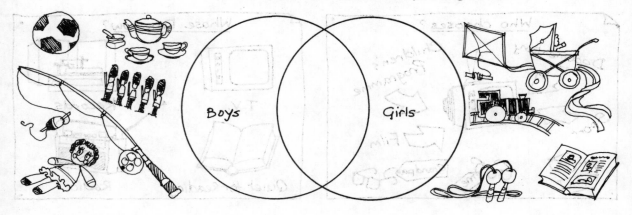

Using diagrams similar to the one shown opposite, ask the children to sort toys, games, activities or jobs into those which they see as specifically for boys, those for girls and those which either might claim.

Are there rules we must obey at home?

If appropriate, reintroduce the topic of rules – this time as they apply to family life. When we belong to a family there are many advantages we enjoy – home, warmth, food, care, protection, etc. However, there are certain rules that we have to obey. Of obvious concern here are home safety rules, but can the children think of rules concerning their behaviour towards other members of the family? Children could be asked to make their own list of rules.

My own rules
– about cleaning teeth . . .
– about keeping clothes tidy . . .
– about helping at home . . .

 There are very clear links here with Chapter 5 (*Looking after myself*) which offer an excellent opportunity to review some of the ways in which children care for themselves. This section also provides a wider context within which to discuss how children have responsibilities to themselves and to others.

Ultimately our health is closely related to choices and decisions we ourselves make and the whole purpose of this book has been to help teachers clarify, for their children, some of the areas in which decisions and choices can indeed be made.

Resources

Because we see the aims of health education and education itself to be so exactly matched, it follows that most children's books can be used in the context of work on 'health'. This includes materials that will be used regularly in the classroom, for example the books in any reading scheme. The books, films, slides, etc mentioned below are therefore only a small selection from the many useful resources available and teachers will no doubt build up their own selection of materials which they find are especially suitable for their own class or group. We would also draw attention to two television series, *Alive and Kicking* (6–7) and *Good Health* (8–11), developed alongside the Project and produced by ATV. Individual programmes are listed in the relevant resource sections below.

We have included a small number of materials which are out of print or no longer available. We have done this where we felt that the material was well known and would be found already in a large number of schools. Failing this, teachers would almost certainly be able to borrow such items from their local library, teachers centre, etc. What we were concerned to do was to point out the relevance of such materials to work on health.

The resources are grouped under chapter headings although there will, of course, be much overlap between these groups. There is a general section at the end, pointing out books that are relevant to work on all aspects of health education.

NOTE
Teachers are reminded that most Area Health Authorities now provide a Health Education service. This service is

normally run by **Health Education Officers** and generally includes advisory services; the supply of certain free materials; the loan of books, films, filmstrips, and models; help with in-service training courses and so-on. We would urge teachers to consult with their local Health Education Officers whose names and addresses may be found by contacting the area offices of the Area Health Authority: see under 'Health Authority' in alphabetical telephone directories. Teachers might also find useful the following publications: *Books for children 5–8: an annotated bibliography with relevance to health education; Teaching aids for children 5–8: an annotated list with relevance to health education*. These are available free of charge from *The Health Education Council*, 78 New Oxford Street, London WC1A 1AH.

1 Finding out about myself

Reference books for teachers

The many human senses by Robert Froman (Bell, 1969)
Penguin primary project: Your body, teacher's handbook by Ted Osborn (Penguin, 1972)
The body by Anthony Smith (Penguin, 1970)
Know your own mind by H. J. Walton (BMA, 1973)

Books and pamphlets for classroom and library

The following series, already familiar to most teachers, will be particularly useful for work on chapter 1, *Finding out about myself: Penguin primary project – Keeping Track* by Sylvia Caveney, *Large as Life* by Gill Evans, *Look What I've Made* by Geoffrey Summerfield; many titles in the Macdonald *Starters* series; *The Human Body* series by Kathleen Elgin (Franklin Watts, 1970); the *Breakthrough* series by David Mackay (Penguin); the *Five Senses* series by Constance Milburn (Blackie, 1975); the '*Mr*' series by Roger Hargreaves (Fabbri); *Use Your Senses* series by Kathleen A. Shoesmith (Burke, 1973); many titles in the *Minibooks* series, the *Beginning Beginner* and the *Beginner* series (Collins). *Discovering Me* and *Discovering You* by Felicia Law (Collins, 1974)
Touch by Arthur Nicholls (Studio Vista, 1975)

How your body works by G. B. B. and Shirley Thomas (Hulton Educational, 1964)

The following deal specifically with the subject of handicap:
Rachel by Elizabeth Fanshawe (Bodley Head, 1975)
Mark's Wheelchair Adventures by Camilla Jessel (Methuen, 1975)

Films, filmstrips, TV and slides

The following are from the *Penguin primary project*:
Insides
Film; 8mm or Filmloop; Super 8mm
Using film taken through x-rays and microscopes.
Outsides
Film; 8mm or Filmloop; Super 8mm
Things people can do using their bodies as a kind of tool or instrument, such as dancing, pole vaulting and tree felling.
The way I feel today
Filmstrip; 35mm; 32 frames
Ways in which we use our bodies, especially in expressing feelings.
Alive and Kicking: Emma and John (ATV) This ITV schools programme is also available as a 16mm colour film from the Rank Film Library. A day in the life of two small children, intended for discussion and relevant to all seven chapters of this Guide. Parts of the film are included in programmes 1–4 of *Alive and Kicking*, while programme 5 repeats it in its entirety. 15 minutes.

Records and cassettes

Heartbeats and mouth music
Record; 33½rpm; 18cm; 16 minutes
(Also from the *Penguin primary project: Your Body*)

Other teaching aids

Know your body (Reeves)
Puzzle; 51 × 29cm; 34 coloured pieces with background. Reeves 'Learn as you play'. Each piece fits into basic human outline with numbers relating to text which explains workings of the organs.

2 How did I begin?

Reference books for teachers

Education for Sexuality: Concepts and Programs for Teaching by John J. Burt and Linda Brower Meeks (W. B. Saunders, 1975)

Sex education in primary school by Albert G. Chanter (Macmillan, 1966)

Peter and Caroline: a child asks about childbirth and sex by Sten Hegeler (Tavistock Publications, 1967)

Learning about Life by Mary Lane (Evans Brothers Limited, 1973)

Sex education: Rationale and Reaction edited by Rex S. Rogers (Cambridge University Press, 1974)

Sex in the childhood years: guidance for parents, counsellors and teachers edited by Isadore Rubin and Lester Kirkendall (Fontana, 1971)

Sexual behaviour of young people by Michael Schofield (Penguin, 1970)

The Body by Anthony Smith (Penguin)

Books and pamphlets for classroom and library

By ensuring that children have ready access to books dealing with human reproduction and sexuality, the teacher helps the development in children of a wholesome attitude to themselves and their bodies. The use of books is a great help in trying to encourage the use of a more public and common language when discussing sexual reproduction.

A baby in our family by Althea Braithwaite (Dinosaur, 1975)

Dan Berry's new baby by Anthony Jones (Blackie, 1969)

How a baby is made by Perholm Knudsen (Pan, 1975)

Where we came from by Mary Lane (Holmes McDougall, 1975)

Where do babies come from? by Margaret Sheffield (Cape, 1973)

How you began by Lennart Nilsson (Keshmi Books, 1975)

How you are made by Christine Palmgen (Dent, 1972)

How you began by Hilary Spiers (Dent, 1971)

All About You: the facts of life explained for younger children (Family Circle, 1969)

Films, filmstrips, TV and slides

How babies are born (Eothen Films)
Film; 16mm; sound; 10 minutes; colour

Animated cartoon film designed to introduce the concepts of both animal and human reproduction.

Merry go round (BBC, 1976)

Film; 16mm; colour

Three films each of 20 minutes: *Beginning*; *Birth*; *Full Circle*. Carefully explained facts of life using cats, dogs, chickens and humans. Includes live births of kittens and human baby; project work for children. Planned for 8–10-year olds.

Where do babies come from? (BBC 1970 – Radio vision series) Radio vision programmes consist of a film strip of 35mm transparencies and a tape recording of a radio broadcast. The two are used simultaneously. The programme aims to give young children factual information about conception and birth.

Alive and Kicking: Looking After Young (ATV) Young wild animals, zoo animals, pets and human beings all need food, sleep, love and attention. 15 minutes. ITV school programme.

Alive and Kicking: On the Farm 1 and 2 (ATV) Part 1 shows the increasing responsibilities (at school and on the farm) of the farmer's children as they grow older. Part 2 stresses the need for cleanliness, regular care and attention when looking after farm animals. Two 15-minute ITV school programmes.

3 What is growing?

Reference books for teachers

Look at kids by Leila Berg (Penguin, 1972)

Sex education in primary school by Albert G. Chanter (Macmillan, 1966)

Your child from five to twelve by R. S. Illingworth (A family doctor booklet, BMA, 1968)

Boys and sex; Girls and sex both by Wardell B. Pomeroy (Penguin, 1970; 1971)

The language of primary school children by Connie and Harold Rosen (Penguin Education for the Schools Council, 1973)

Books and pamphlets for classroom and library

This subject lends itself particularly well to fantasy and humour and there is much material available to support this treatment. Hilaire Belloc's cautionary verses, for example, would be appropriate.

Tony's hard work day by Alan Arkin (Andre Deutsch, 1975)
Titch by Pat Hutchins (Penguin, 1974)
Flat Stanley (a play adapted from the story by Jeff Brown) by
    Sheila Lane and Marion Kemp (Penguin Education, 1972)
Peter's chair by Ezra Jack Keats (Penguin, 1973)

Children's story books provide opportunities for children to explore, recognize and cope with emotions – both their own and other people's. Teachers should take advantage of such opportunities of exploring this important side of growing – emotional growth.

Films, filmstrips, TV and slides

Good Health: Everybody's Different (ATV) Emphasizes that we all grow in skills as well as in size and that as we grow we must learn to make more decisions and take more responsibility. 15 minutes. An ITV schools programme, also available as a 16mm colour film from Rank Film Library.

Other teaching aids

Across the generations – a first pack for primary schools.
(*Help the Aged* Education Department, 1975)
Portfolio: Five 'read and think' cards; two work cards; three sets of story cards; story book; poetry sheet; four photographs; book list; teacher's notes.

4 What helps me grow?

Reference books for teachers

Attachment by John Bowlby (Penguin, 1971)
Child care and the growth of love by John Bowlby and
    Margaret Fry (Penguin, 1970)
*Food and nutrition education in the primary school: A guide
    for its introduction* produced by the Food and Agricultural
    Organization of the United Nations (H.M.S.O., 1971)
Play with a purpose for under-sevens by Elizabeth M.
Matterson (Penguin, 1965)

The Psychology of Play by Susanna Miller (Penguin, 1968)
   The child's discovery of space – from hopscotch to mazes : an introduction to intuitive topology by Jean and Simonne Sauvy (Penguin, 1974)

Books and pamphlets for classroom and library

As we saw on page 47, it is important to include discussions of love and care when considering *What helps me grow?* The following books can provide starting points for such discussions:

George and the baby by Althea Braithwaite (Dinosaur Publications, 1973)
The new baby by Althea Braithwaite (Souvenir Press, 1973)
Love is a special way of feeling by Joan Walsh Anglund (Collins, 1960)
What colour is love? by Joan Walsh Anglund (Collins, 1967)
My home and yours by Peggy Blakely (Black, 1971)
Your children need you (a *Health Education Council* leaflet)
God bless love : a collection of children's sayings compiled by Nanette Newman (Collins, 1972)

Books which cover the topics of exercise, rest and food, and their importance in helping growth:

About the vegetables on your plate by Vera Elwell Allee and Isadro de la Rosa (Frederich Muller, 1965)
The sleep factory by Norman Daymil (Fabbri, 1974)
Dog so small by Philippa Pearce (Penguin, 1970)
Sleep book by Dr. Seuss (Collins, 1964)
Sleep is for everyone by Paul Showers (A. & C. Black, 1974)
The 'Food' section of the *Penguin primary project* will be useful for work on this chapter.

Films, filmstrips, TV and slides

Busy Bodies (USA Stanton Films, 1969; Hadleigh: Boulton-Hawker Films)
Film; 16mm; Sound; 10 minutes; colour
Sleep heads (USA Stanton Films, 1964; Hadleigh: Boulton-Hawker Films)
Film; 16mm; sound; 10 minutes; colour
You and your food (Walt Disney, 1955)
Film; 16mm; sound; 8 minutes; colour
Alive and Kicking: Movement (ATV) A model skeleton shows how bones make movement possible. Physical education

sequences demonstrate how training improves performance. 15 minutes. ITV schools programme.

Alive and Kicking: Keeping Well (ATV) The human body is compared to an old car: both need fuel, care, attention and periods of rest if they are to function properly. 15 minutes. ITV schools programme.

Good Health: Exercise and Rest (ATV) Children demonstrate how muscles and bones work, and the need for sleep. 15 minutes. ITV schools programme, also available as a 16mm colour film from Rank Film Library.

Records and cassettes

The following are all from the *Penguin primary project*:
Bread
Record; 33½rpm; 18cm
Traditional song, *John Barleycorn*, interspersed with narrative from modern farmers, grain dealers and millers on the story of wheat.
Eating away
Record; 33½rpm; 18cm
A collection of food experiences, for example how a Nigerian feels about food in England, a cameraman's story of food in the Amazon territory, and eating in prison.
Working and Dancing
Record; 33½rpm; 18cm
Musical expressions of people around the world in backbreaking or monotonous labour or in celebration, i.e. pounding grain in Malawi, shrinking tweed in the Hebrides and Jamaican Reggae.
Food table: a sun, soil, plant and animal food chain
Film; 8mm or Super 8mm; Silent; 4 minutes; colour

Other teaching aids

Numerous charts, cards, games etc, are produced on food and nutrition. The following organizations produce a number of teaching aids: *British Diabetic Association; Kelloggs Education Department; National Dairy Council; Heinz Home Cookery Service.*

5 Looking after myself

Reference books for teachers

The young smoker : a study of smoking among schoolboys carried out for the Ministry of Health by J. M. Bynner (H.M.S.O., 1969)

Care of the feet (Consumers Association, 1975)

Caring for teeth (Consumers Association, 1970)

Man against disease by A. G. Clegg and P. Catherine (Heinemann Educational Books, 1973)

Out of the mouths by H. Colin Davis and Doreen Land (Gibbs Oral Hygiene Service)

Health and disease by Rene Dubos and Maya Pines (Time-Life International, 1969)

Man, Medicine and Environment by Rene Dubos (Penguin, 1970)

Disease and world health by Nance Lui Fyson (Batsford, 1973)

Children's footwear – the report of the Committee appointed by the Chancellor of the Exchequer (H.M.S.O., 1973)

Man, Environment and Disease in Britain – a medical geography of Britain through the ages by George Melvyn Howe (David and Charles, 1972)

Planning teaching about drugs, alcohol and cigarettes (I.S.D.D., 1974)

Understanding medicine by Roger James (Penguin, 1970)

Children's dental health in England and Wales (1973) by J. E. Todd (H.M.S.O., 1975)

Books and pamphlets for classroom and library

There are a number of books and series which will help in allaying children's fears of doctors, dentists and hospitals. For example, the *Topsy and Tim* series by Jean and Gareth Adamson (Blackie); *Going into hospital, Going to the doctor,* and *Visiting the dentist* by Althea Braithwaite (Dinosaur); *Children's hospital colouring book* (Nawch); *Simon goes to hospital* (Nawch); several titles in the 'Sparks' series (Blackie); *Doctor and the nurse* by J. T. Francis and F. J. Ashworth (Holmes McDougall, 1973); *My Doctor* by Harlow Rochwell (Hamish Hamilton, 1974); *The Nurse* by Vera Southgate (Ladybird Books, Wills and Hepworth, 1963).

There are many publications, pamphlets, etc produced on

the subject of dental health. Organizations which produce materials for children include the *General Dental Council, Gibbs Oral Hygiene Service,* The *Health Education Council* and *Area Health Authorities.* Of particular interest are the following publications:

Published by *Gibbs Oral Hygiene Service*:

Brushing your teeth; Your mouth is a living machine by Colin H. Davis

Finding out about the brighter smile (a *Tramline* project book): *Teddy and Belinda* by Elsie B. Mills; *The sad story of a tooth.*

Fleas by Joanna Cole (World's Work, 1973)

Your Body by David Scott Daniell (Ladybird books, Wills and Hepworth, 1967)

Health and disease – Macdonald First Library (Macdonald Educational, 1974)

The Story of Medicine by Edmund Hunter (Ladybird books, Wills and Hepworth, 1972)

Once there was a river : a story of water pollution by Elenore T. Pounds (Scott Foresman, 1974)

Clothes children wore by Peter Rice (Dinosaur, 1974)

Clothes by Vera Southgate (Macmillan, 1968)

Emma and the measles by Gunilla Wolde (Brockhampton Press, 1975)

Harry the dirty dog by Gene Zion (Penguin, 1968)

There are also a number of publications dealing with foot care. For example: *Jane and Miranda* – a family doctor booklet (B.M.A., 1970); *Six Important Shoe Facts for Foot Health* – a bookmark (Health Education Council); *Start-Rite Stay Right* (Start-Rite Shoes).

Films, filmstrips, TV and slides

Dentist (Hounslow Department of Health, 1973; London: B.M.A. Film Library)

Film; 16mm; sound; 5 minutes; colour

A young boy visits the dentist for a routine inspection and the equipment and procedures are explained to him.

Good Health: White Ivory (ATV) A dentist and children demonstrate what happens if teeth are not brushed properly. 15 minutes. ITV schools programme, also available as a 16mm colour film from Rank Film Library.

Good Health: Talking Feet (ATV) A film made in a junior

school about a strike organized by feet who complain that they are not being properly treated. 15 minutes. ITV schools programme, also available as a 16mm colour film from Rank Film Library.

Good Health: Germs, Germs, Germs (ATV) A junior school's portrayal of the different ways in which germs attack human beings. 15 minutes. ITV schools programme, also available as a 16mm colour film from Rank Film Library.

Alive and Kicking: Clothing (ATV) Police drivers and speedway racers show the protective nature of clothing. 15 minutes. ITV schools programme.

Take care of your teeth (Educational Productions) Filmstrip; 24 single frames; Black and white

Posters and charts

Both the *General Dental Council* and *Gibbs Oral Hygiene Service* produce a number of useful charts and posters.

Be a womble (Keep Britain Tidy Group)
76 × 51cm; colour

A beautiful world – don't spoil it (Blue Peter/Keep Britain Tidy)
76 × 51cm; colour; (Designed by a seven-year-old)

Keep Britain Tidy! (Keep Britain Tidy Group)
76 × 51cm or 38 × 25cm; colour

Keep flu to yourself (Health Education Council)
77 × 51cm; black and white

Such small rubbish . . . but it can kill! (Blue Peter/Keep Britain Tidy)
76 × 50cm; (Designed by a twelve-year-old)

Your country, your problem – litter (Keep Britain Tidy Group)
38 × 26cm; colour

Other teaching aids

The foot health pack (Clarks Buckinghamshire Chiropody and Health Education Section)
10 wall charts and 6 sets of work cards. Work cards are linked to charts. Includes notes for teachers (24p).

I'm a womble. I Keep Britain Tidy (Keep Britain Tidy Group)
Button; 6cm; colour

Keep Britain tidy (Keep Britain Tidy Group)

Button; 6cm; colour
Illustrated with Walt Disney's Mickey Mouse and Minnie.
Keep Britain Tidy (Keep Britain Tidy Group)
White T-shirt with illustration
Donald Duck *or* Mickey Mouse and Minnie Mouse.
*Health and safety nightlights: pictures and songs for young
children* by Elenore T. Pounds (Scott Foresman, 1970)
Record; 33½rpm; 25cm; Portfolio; 38 × 47cm; 12 coloured
pieces
Photographic charts of children in activities such as washing
hands, crossing the street, getting weighed and measured.
Teachers resource booklet. Intended for four- and five-year-
olds.

6 Keeping safe

Reference books for teachers

Safety for your family by Angela Creese (Mills and Boon,
1974)

Books and pamphlets for classroom and library

Teachers should take advantage of all opportunities to talk
about safety, many of which will occur when reading stories.
The *Topsy and Tim* series, already mentioned on page 128
will be useful in connection with work on safety, in particular
the titles *Topsy and Tim go safely*; *Topsy and Tim learn to
swim*; *Topsy and Tim take no risks*. Several titles in the *Our
friends at work* series (Holmes McDougall) are useful.
Don't Panic by Audry Coppard (Heinemann, 1975)
A busy road by Elizabeth Goodacre (Blackie, 1971)

Films, filmstrips, TV and slides

How to have an accident in the home (Walt Disney, 1956)
Film; 16mm; sound; 8 minutes; colour
Road safety – between parked cars (Educational Productions,
1973)
Filmstrip; 36 double frames; colour
Alive and Kicking: Safety (ATV) Topics include the dangers
of water play, guide dog safety training and crossing the
road. 15 minutes. ITV schools programme.

Posters and charts

The *Royal Society for the Prevention of Accidents* (ROSPA) produces a number of useful posters and charts.
Look for the kitemark (British Standards Institution; Consumer Standards Advisory Committee)
44 × 32cm; black and white

Other teaching aids

Environmental studies worksheets by B. G. Jolly and P. Goodsell (Collins, 1971)
Each pack contains 20 worksheets together with teachers' notes.
My town: shops, roads, flats and houses to help me find my way. (ESA Creative Learning, 1974)
41 pieces
Shaped wooden blocks representing buildings, streets and parks. A Susan Wynter toy.

7 Knowing about others

Reference books for teachers

Discovery of death in childhood and after by Sylvia Anthony (Penguin, 1973)
Education for a change: community action and the school by Colin and Meg Ball (Penguin, 1973)
Other worlds edited by Donald Ball – *Penguin English Project stage one* (Penguin, 1971)
Violence in human society by John Gunn (David and Charles, 1973)
Family and kinship in east London by Michael Young and Peter Willmott (Penguin, 1962)

Books and pamphlets for classroom and library

A list of books that could be used in connection with work on this chapter would be an endless one. Certainly all children's story books are relevant and indeed story telling can form a basis for discussion, role-playing and drama as well as written work. By pinpointing characters' attitudes towards and feelings about each other, teachers help develop in children an understanding leading to social awareness and responsibility.

Bad boys edited by Eileen H. Colwell (Penguin, 1972)

James and the giant peach by Roald Dahl (Penguin, 1973)

Patchwork grandmother by Nance Donkin (Hamish Hamilton, 1975)

Very naughty little sister by Dorothy Edwards (Penguin, 1970)

A wet monday by Dorothy Edwards (Methuen, 1975)

Happy lion by Louise Fatio (Penguin, 1970)

Family from One End Street by Eve Garnett (Penguin, 1971)

Trouble with Jack by Shirley Hughes (Collins, 1973)

When Violet died by Mildred Kantrowitz and Emily A. McCulley (Bodley Head, 1974)

Peter's chair by Ezra Jack Keats (Penguin, 1973)

The Hollyport family by Margaret Kornitzer (Bodley Head, 1973)

I am adopted by Susan Lapsley (Bodley Head, 1974)

Don't Forget Tom by Hanne Larsen (A. & C. Black, 1974)

May I bring a friend? by Beatrice Regniers (Penguin, 1972)

My family by Felicity Sen (Bodley Head, 1975)

Hundred and one Dalmatians by Dodie Smith (Penguin, 1969)

A taste of blackberries by Doris Buchanan Smith (Heinemann, 1975)

Elephant and the bad baby by Efrida Vipont and Raymond Briggs (Penguin, 1971)

Adventures of the little wooden horse by Ursula Moray Williams (Penguin, 1970)

Different Peter and Emma ; Emma and the measles ; Emma's baby brother – all by Gunilla Wolde (Brockhampton Press, 1974)

George and the baby by Althea Braithwaite (Dinosaur, 1973)

The new baby by Althea Braithwaite (Souvenir, 1973)

A friend is someone who likes you by Ivan Walsh Anglund (Collins, 1959)

Helping at home by M. Gagg (Ladybird Books, Willis and Hepworth, 1968)

Mummy's health visitor by Anita Harper (Blackie, 1973)

Alive Alive-o (Book 1) by Zorwert P. Jones and S. F. Jex (Blond Educational, 1968)

Discovering me and discovering you by Felicia Law (Collins, 1974)

What do people do all day? by Richard Scarry (Collins, 1968)

Films, filmstrips, TV and slides

Hopscotch (USA Churchill, 1972; Ipswich: Boulton-Hawker)
Film; 16mm; 12 minutes; colour
Whimsical, animated story about an eager but socially inept
little boy and his many attempts to win the friendship of
two children. Sound but no narration.
Good Health: One of the Family (ATV) The story of an
eight-year-old boy who suffers from spina bifida and how his
family helps to look after him. 15 minutes. ITV schools
programme, also available as a 16mm colour film from Rank
Film Library.

Records and cassettes

The following two records are from the *Penguin primary
project*:
Families round the world
Record; 33½rpm; 18cm
Songs which illustrate some of the ways people celebrate
important family events in different parts of the world.
Families song and dance
Record; 33½rpm; 18cm
Folk songs and games that tell you something about families
– about choosing a husband or wife, having children, getting
old and dying.

Other teaching aids

Families game (Penguin, 1974)
Cardsets – 150 cards in 6 sets
To involve children in identification with specific aspects
of family life by means of dramatic activity and role-playing.

General

Reference books for teachers

*Anatomy of Judgement: investigation into the processes of
  perception and reasoning* by Minnie Louie Johnson
  Abercrombie (Penguin, 1969)
School that I'd Like by Edward Blishen (Penguin, 1969)

Children in Distress (second edition) by Sir Alec Clegg and Barbara Megson (Penguin, 1973)

A textbook of health education for students in colleges of education, teachers and health educators by A. J. Dalzell-Ward (Tavistock Publications, 1974)

A handbook of Health Education issued by the Department of Education and Science (H.M.S.O., 1968)

Health Education in Schools – report of the working party issued by the Scottish Education Department (H.M.S.O., 1974)

Health Education index and guide to voluntary social welfare organisations by B. Edsall

Education and the working class by Brian Jackson and Dennis Marsden (Penguin, 1966)

Family and School edited by David Jackson (Penguin, 1970)

Male and Female by Margaret Mead (Penguin, 1964)

The child under stress by Edna Oakshott (Priory Press, 1973)

Health Science and the young child by Marion B. Pollock and Delbert Oberteuffer (Harper and Row, 1974)

School curriculum by Kenneth W. Richmond (Methuen, 1971)

Teaching elementary health science by Walter D. Sorochan and Stephen J. Bender (Addison-Wesley, 1975)

Junior Voices: an anthology of poetry and pictures (Books 1–4) edited by Geoffrey Summerfield (Penguin)

Education, the child and society – a documentary history 1900–1973 edited by William van der Eyken (Penguin, 1973)

Teaching health in elementary schools by Maryhelen Vannier (Lea and Fibirger, 1974)

Health Education in the elementary school by Carl E. Willgoose (W. B. Saunders, 1974)

Children under stress by Sula Wolff (Penguin, 1973)

Books and pamphlets for classroom and library

Health and growth (Books 1–4) by J. B. Richmond (Scott, Foresman)

Films, filmstrips and slides

Development by feelings in children (USA: Parents Magazine; Beckenham: Edward Patterson Associates)
Film; 16mm; sound; 35 minutes; colour

Television Programmes

A number of programmes in the ATV series *Alive and Kicking* and *Good Health* have been listed above. Other programmes in the *Good Health* series are available, but may be found more suitable for older children. Teachers are advised to consult ITV and BBC annual programme booklets for details of these and other individual programmes which may prove useful, and for programme showing times.